Cookir

HEALTHY HEART

recipes · hints · tips

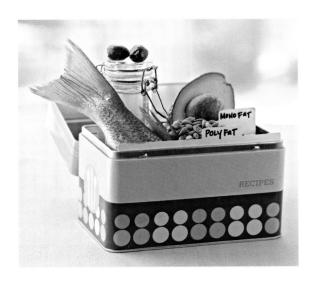

Oxmoor
House®

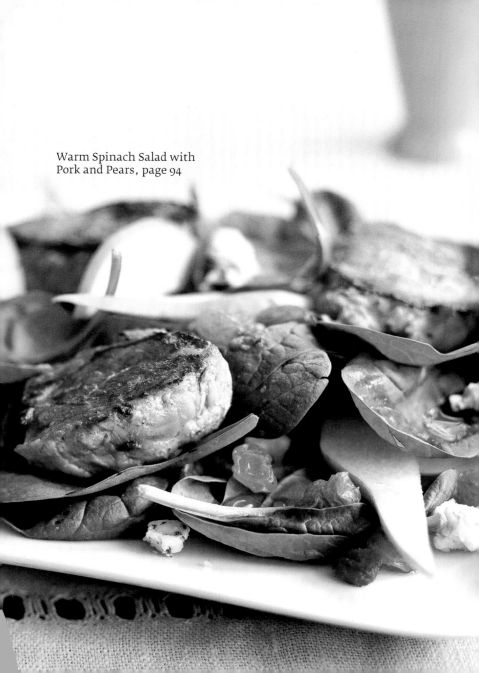

Warm Spinach Salad with
Pork and Pears, page 94

Welcome

Most heart health–conscious cooks today want to prepare delicious meals that their friends and family will rave about. That's why we've created *Cooking Light Eat Smart Guide: Healthy Heart*. With more than 70 sure-to-please recipes, you'll find the keys to crafting flavorful, good-for-you dishes over and over again.

If you're feeling confused and overwhelmed about how to select and prepare heart-healthy foods for your loved ones, then let *Cooking Light Eat Smart Guide: Healthy Heart* help you plan meals without having to wonder, "Is this really good for us?" Offering more than just recipes, this handy go-to guide is jam-packed with quick answers for those who are seeking practical advice for heart health–related shopping, cooking, and eating.

Chock-full of mouthwatering and wholesome options, this book offers a wide array of simple entrées, refreshing salads, filling soups, sensational sandwiches, and decadent desserts. Every recipe has been tested at least twice to ensure quality and satisfaction. In addition, each recipe comes with a complete nutrition analysis to help you make savvy choices that suit your lifestyle.

Cooking Light Eat Smart Guide: Healthy Heart gives you the tools necessary to make preparing heart-smart dishes easier and more delicious than ever before. We hope this cookbook will bring exciting new possibilities to your cooking repertoire and that you will discover how effortless it can be to make heart-healthy foods taste great!

The *Cooking Light* Editors

ISBN-13: 978-0-8487-3305-6
ISBN-10: 0-8487-3305-3
Library of Congress Control Number: 2009937182
Printed in the United States of America
First printing 2010

Be sure to check with your health-care provider before making any changes in your diet.

OXMOOR HOUSE

VP, Publishing Director: Jim Childs
Editorial Director: Susan Payne Dobbs
Brand Manager: Michelle Turner Aycock
Senior Editor: Heather Averett
Managing Editor: Laurie S. Herr

Cooking Light Eat Smart Guide: Healthy Heart

Editor: Andrea C. Kirkland, M.S., R.D.
Project Editor: Diane Rose
Senior Designer: Emily Albright Parrish
Director, Test Kitchens: Elizabeth Tyler Austin
Assistant Director, Test Kitchens:
  Julie Christopher
Test Kitchens Professionals:
  Allison E. Cox, Julie Gunter,
  Kathleen Royal Phillips,
  Catherine Crowell Steele,
  Ashley T. Strickland
Photography Director: Jim Bathie
Senior Photo Stylist: Kay E. Clarke
Associate Photo Stylist:
  Katherine Eckert Coyne
Production Manager: Theresa Beste-Farley

Contributors

Compositor: Teresa Cole
Copy Editor: Rhonda Richards
Interns: Christine T. Boatwright,
  Georgia Dodge, Caitlin Watzke

To order additional publications, call 1-800-765-6400 or 1-800-491-0551.

For more books to enrich your life, visit **oxmoorhouse.com**

To search, savor, and share thousands of recipes, visit **myrecipes.com**

Cooking Light

Editor: Scott Mowbray
Creative Director: Carla Frank
Deputy Editor: Phillip Rhodes
Food Editor: Ann Taylor Pittman
Special Publications Editor:
  Mary Simpson Creel, M.S., R.D.
Nutrition Editor: Kathy Kitchens Downie, R.D.
Associate Food Editors: Timothy Q. Cebula,
  Julianna Grimes
Associate Editors: Cindy Hatcher,
  Brandy Rushing
Test Kitchen Director: Vanessa T. Pruett
Assistant Test Kitchen Director:
  Tiffany Vickers Davis
Chief Food Stylist: Charlotte Fekete
Senior Food Stylist: Kellie Gerber Kelley
Recipe Testers and Developers:
  Robin Bashinsky, Adam Hickman,
  Deb Wise
Art Director: Fernande Bondarenko
Junior Deputy Art Director:
  Alexander Spacher
Designer: Chase Turberville
Photo Director: Kristen Schaefer
Senior Photographer: Randy Mayor
Senior Photo Stylist: Cindy Barr
Photo Stylist: Leigh Ann Ross
Copy Chief: Maria Parker Hopkins
Assistant Copy Chief: Susan Roberts
Research Editor: Michelle Gibson Daniels
Editorial Production Director: Liz Rhoades
Production Editor: Hazel R. Eddins
Art/Production Assistant: Josh Rutledge
Administrative Coordinator: Carol D. Johnson
CookingLight.com Editor: Allison Long Lowery
CookingLight.com Nutrition Editor:
  Holley Johnson Grainger, M.S., R.D.
CookingLight.com Production Assistant:
  Mallory Daugherty

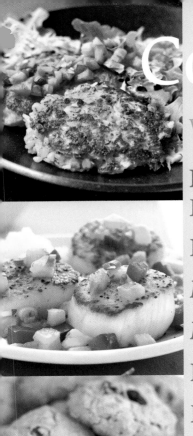

Contents

Heart-Smart Basics

Find out what you need to know about eating a heart-healthy diet. Follow these basic guidelines, and you'll be on your way to optimum heart health.

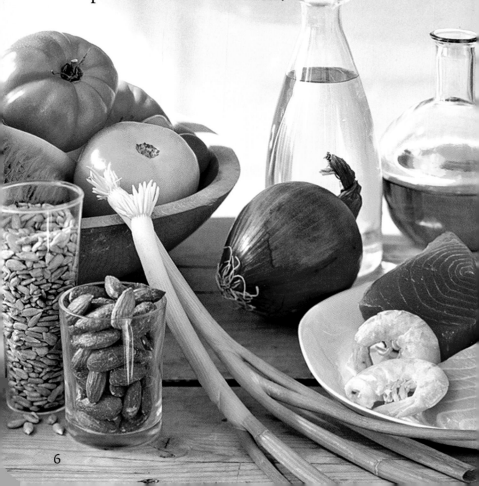

Be calorie conscious to control your weight.

Weight control is important in the prevention and treatment of heart disease. Excess weight makes the heart work harder, causing increased blood pressure. It also raises blood cholesterol and triglyceride levels and lowers HDL ("good") cholesterol. A modest weight loss of at least 10 pounds has been shown to decrease a person's risk for heart disease as well as diabetes.

To maintain a healthy weight, balance calories from foods and beverages with calories expended. The secret to this delicate balance is knowing how to determine adequate portion sizes. The United States Department of Agriculture's MyPyramid provides general healthy-eating guidelines and includes recommendations for portion sizes of different foods. Available online, the interactive pyramid allows users to tailor it to their needs based on age, gender, height, weight, and activity levels. Check it out at **www.mypyramid.gov**.

Know your fats.

Here's what you need to know about fitting fats into your diet.

MONOUNSATURATED FATS Liquid at room temperature, these plant-based fats can lower cholesterol when used in place of saturated fat in the diet.
Sources: Canola, olive, and peanut oils; peanuts; pecans; and avocados.

POLYUNSATURATED FATS These plant- and fish-derived fats can lower cholesterol when they replace saturated fat in the diet. Fatty fish such as salmon and tuna contain omega-3 fatty acids, a group of polyunsaturated fats that keep the heart healthy, even when consumed in small amounts.
Sources: Vegetable oils such as safflower, sunflower, soybean, corn, and sesame oils; sunflower seeds; soybeans; fatty fish such as tuna, mackerel, and salmon; and most nuts.

(continued)

SATURATED FATS Concentrated mostly in animal products, these solid fats raise harmful LDL cholesterol and increase the risk of cardiovascular disease.
Sources: Beef, lamb, pork, bacon, cheese, full-fat yogurt, butter, and whole milk. Snack chips and bakery items made with tropical oils such as coconut, palm, and palm kernel also contain these fats, which are solid at room temperature.

The key with saturated fats is to choose wisely and use them in moderation. For example, use only small amounts of cheese to heighten a dish's flavor, or make vegetables the main feature of the dish rather than meat. If you eat red meat as a main course, stick to the recommended serving size—3 ounces, or about the size of a deck of cards on your plate. For dairy products, choosing 1% or fat-free options helps limit the amount of saturated fat in your diet.

TRANS FATS Produced when liquid oils are processed into solid shortenings, trans fats (also known as partially hydrogenated oils) raise LDL ("bad") cholesterol and lower HDL ("good") cholesterol.
Sources: Foods can harbor trans fats if they're made with partially hydrogenated oils. Since January 2006, the Food and Drug Administration has required all food manufacturers to indicate the amount of trans fat in a serving of food. (Food with less than one-half gram of trans fat per serving can be labeled "trans fat–free.") Some meat and dairy products contain trace amounts of naturally occurring trans fats. It's unknown whether these fats have the same harmful effects on your health as manufactured trans fats.

Slash sodium.

For most people, the more sodium you consume, the higher your blood pressure will be. And as blood pressure jumps, so does the risk for heart disease and stroke. The American Heart Association recommends limiting sodium to 1,500 milligrams per day.

Go for whole grains.

Research shows that eating just 2½ servings of whole grains per day is enough to lower your risk for heart disease. (One serving equals a slice of 100% whole-wheat bread or ⅓ cup cooked brown rice.) And it appears that greater whole-grain intake is associated with a decreased risk of obesity, diabetes, high blood pressure, and high cholesterol.

Focus on healthy foods, and strive for variety.

To fight heart disease, the American Heart Association recommends eating an assortment of nutritious foods daily. Make an effort to follow these diet guidelines to get the nutrients your body needs and add variety to your diet.

• Eat at least two 3.5-ounce servings a week of fish, preferably oily fish such as salmon, tuna, or mackerel.

• Consume at least 4 servings of nuts, legumes, and seeds a week.

• Select fiber-rich whole grains and consume at least 3 servings a day.

• Limit sugar-sweetened beverages to no more than 450 calories (36 ounces) a week.

• Limit processed meats to no more than 2 servings a week.

• Limit saturated fat and trans fat to less than 7% and 1%, respectively, of total energy intake.

• Choose fruits and vegetables in all the colors of the rainbow—be sure to eat at least 4½ cups a day.

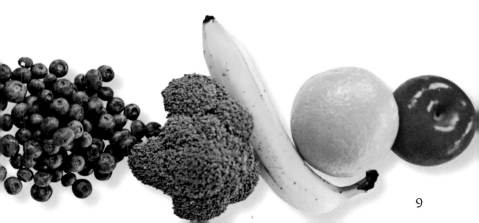

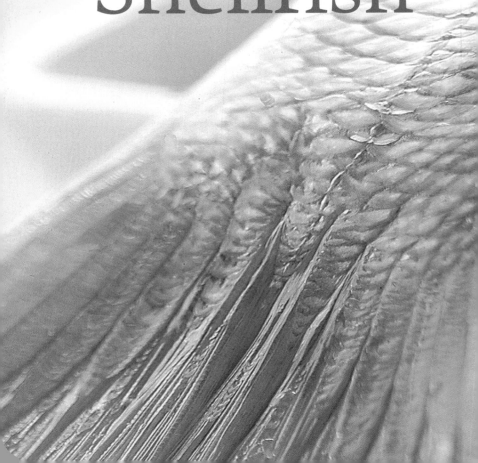

HEALTHY HEART

Fish & Shellfish

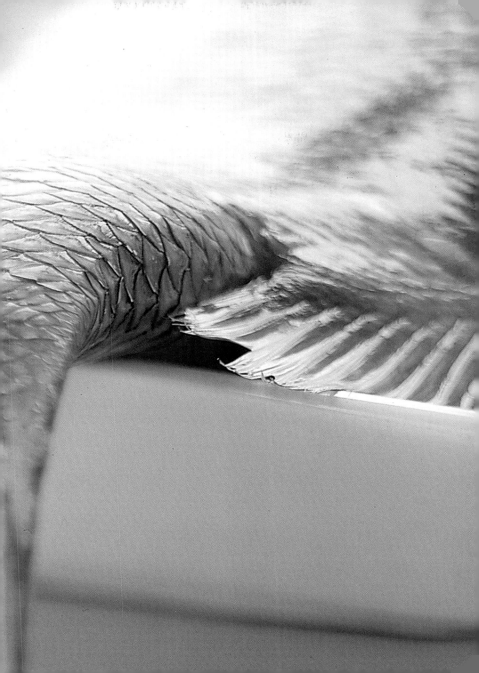

QUICK&EASY

Pistachio-Crusted Grouper with Lavender Honey Sauce

The delicate, subtle flavors of roasted pistachios and lavender honey transform this baked grouper into an easy yet refined meal that family and friends will remember. Serve with sautéed spinach.

5 tablespoons dry breadcrumbs
5 tablespoons finely chopped unsalted shelled dry-roasted pistachios
4 (6-ounce) grouper fillets
1/4 teaspoon salt
1/4 teaspoon freshly ground black pepper

2 large egg whites, lightly beaten
2 tablespoons butter
2 tablespoons lavender honey
1 tablespoon fresh lemon juice
Lemon wedges (optional)
Lavender sprigs (optional)

1. Preheat oven to 450°.

2. Combine breadcrumbs and pistachios in a shallow dish. Sprinkle fillets evenly with salt and pepper. Dip fillets in egg whites; dredge in breadcrumb mixture.

3. Place fish on a jelly-roll pan lined with parchment paper; bake at 450° for 12 minutes or until fish flakes easily when tested with a fork or until desired degree of doneness.

4. While fish cooks, melt butter in a small saucepan over medium heat. Add honey and lemon juice, stirring to combine. Drizzle fillets evenly with lavender honey sauce. Garnish with lemon wedges and lavender sprigs, if desired. **YIELD:** 4 servings (serving size: 1 fillet and about 1 tablespoon sauce).

CALORIES 337; FAT 12g (sat 4.7g, mono 4.3g, poly 2.3g); PROTEIN 37.7g; CARB 18.1g; FIBER 1.5g; CHOL 78mg; IRON 2.4mg; SODIUM 360mg; CALC 26mg

RECIPE BENEFIT: low-sodium

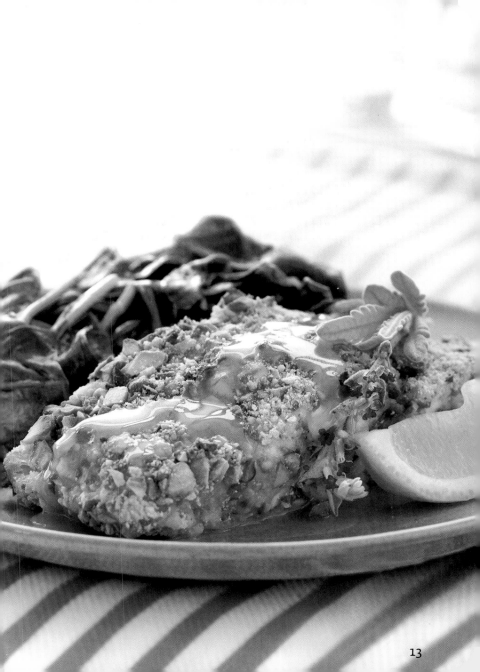

CHOICE INGREDIENT: *Edamame*

Edamame (fresh soybeans) are packed with potential health benefits. Each $\frac{1}{2}$-cup serving contains 4 grams of fiber and only 3 grams of fat, all of which are the heart-healthy mono- and polyunsaturated kind. The beans are also high in soy protein, which may help reduce cholesterol when part of a low-fat diet.

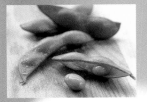

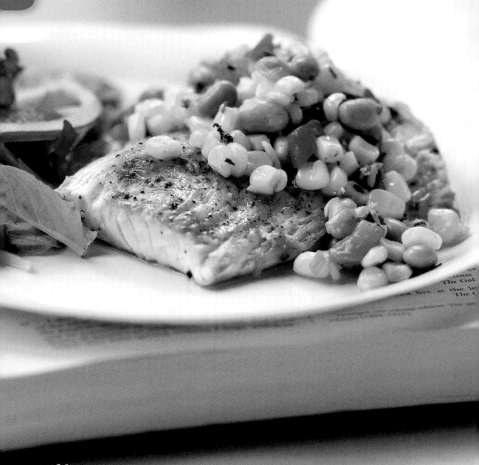

Seared Mahimahi with Edamame Succotash

1 medium red bell pepper	1¹/₃ cups frozen corn kernels, thawed
¹/₄ cup finely chopped green onions	¹/₂ cup frozen shelled edamame (green soybeans), thawed
2 teaspoons chopped fresh thyme	1 teaspoon olive oil
2 teaspoons rice wine vinegar	Cooking spray
2 teaspoons fresh lime juice	4 (6-ounce) mahimahi or other firm white fish fillets
2 teaspoons olive oil	
¹/₄ teaspoon salt	¹/₈ teaspoon salt
¹/₄ teaspoon ground red pepper	¹/₈ teaspoon freshly ground black pepper
2 garlic cloves, minced	

1. Preheat broiler.

2. Cut bell pepper in half lengthwise; discard seeds and membranes. Place pepper halves, skin side up, on a foil-lined baking sheet; flatten with hand. Broil 15 minutes or until blackened. Place in a zip-top plastic bag; seal. Let stand 10 minutes. Peel and finely chop. Combine pepper, onions, and next 7 ingredients, tossing to combine.

3. Combine corn and beans in a small microwave-safe bowl; cover with water. Microwave at HIGH 2 minutes; drain. Add corn mixture to bell pepper mixture; toss to combine.

4. Heat 1 teaspoon oil in a large nonstick skillet coated with cooking spray over medium-high heat. Sprinkle both sides of fish with ¹/₈ teaspoon salt and ¹/₈ teaspoon black pepper. Add fish to pan; cook 4 minutes on each side or until fish flakes easily when tested with a fork. Serve with succotash. YIELD: 4 servings (serving size: 1 fillet and ¹/₂ cup succotash).

CALORIES 379; FAT 9.4g (sat 1.5g, mono 5.5g, poly 1.6g); PROTEIN 35.8g; CARB 41.2g; FIBER 8g; CHOL 52mg; IRON 3.7mg; SODIUM 537mg; CALC 84mg

RECIPE BENEFITS: low-fat; high-fiber

Fish

With the enormous variety of fresh fish available at supermarkets today, you can surely find a fish to suit anyone's palate—from assertive salmon to subtle tilapia, from buttery halibut to meaty tuna and beyond.

BUYING FISH

Often the fresh fish you buy to prepare at home has been frozen. Fish sold as fresh can be anywhere from one day to two weeks out of the water. Large fishing vessels may stay at sea for two weeks, keeping their catch on ice to sell fresh. For top quality, look for "Frozen-at-Sea" (FAS)—fish that has been flash-frozen at extremely low temperatures in as little as 3 seconds onboard ship. When thawed, sea-frozen fish are almost indistinguishable from fresh fish.

WHOLE FRESH FISH

• Look for shiny skin; tightly adhering scales; bright, clear eyes; firm, taut flesh that springs back when pressed; and a moist, flat tail.

• Gills should be cherry-red, not brownish.

• Saltwater fish should smell briny; freshwater fish should smell like a clean pond.

FRESH FILLETS OR STEAKS

• When buying white-fleshed fish, choose translucent-looking fillets with a pinkish tint.

• When buying any color fish, the flesh should appear dense without any gaps between layers.

• If the fish is wrapped in plastic, the package should contain little to no liquid.

• Ask the fishmonger to remove any pin bones, which run crosswise to the backbone.

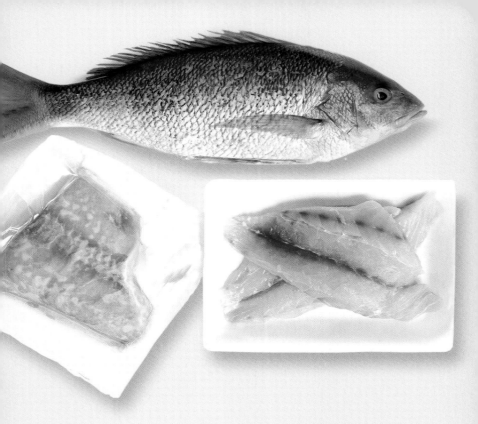

FROZEN FISH
• Look for shiny, rock-hard frozen fish with no white freezer-burn spots, frost, or ice crystals.

• Choose well-sealed packages from the bottom of the freezer case that are at most three months old.

STORING FISH
Buy fish on your way out of the store, take it directly home, and cook (or freeze) it within 24 hours. Keep the fish as cold as possible until you're ready to cook it by storing it in the coldest part of your refrigerator.

QUICK&**EASY**

Sautéed Snapper with Orange-Fennel Salad

The salad brings bright, fresh Mediterranean flavors to this simple fish dish. A mandoline slices fennel evenly.

2	oranges	$^{1}/_{2}$	teaspoon freshly ground black
1	medium fennel bulb with stalks		pepper, divided
2	tablespoons olive oil, divided	4	(6-ounce) red snapper fillets
$^{3}/_{4}$	teaspoon salt, divided	$^{1}/_{2}$	teaspoon fresh thyme leaves

1. Peel and section oranges over a bowl, reserving 2 tablespoons juice. Thinly slice fennel bulb; chop 1 teaspoon fronds. Discard stalks. Place orange sections and sliced fennel in a medium bowl. Combine reserved juice, fronds, 1 tablespoon olive oil, $^{1}/_{4}$ teaspoon salt, and $^{1}/_{4}$ teaspoon freshly ground black pepper in a small bowl, stirring with a whisk. Drizzle juice mixture over fennel mixture; toss well to coat.

2. Heat remaining 1 tablespoon olive oil in a large nonstick skillet over medium-high heat. Sprinkle fish evenly with $^{1}/_{2}$ teaspoon salt, $^{1}/_{4}$ teaspoon freshly ground black pepper, and thyme. Add fish to pan; cook 4 minutes on each side or until desired degree of doneness. Serve with fennel salad. YIELD: 4 servings (serving size: 1 fillet and about $^{1}/_{2}$ cup salad).

CALORIES 283; FAT 9.5g (sat 1.5g, mono 5.8g, poly 1.4g); PROTEIN 36.3g; CARB 12.2g; FIBER 3.4g; CHOL 63mg; IRON 0.8mg; SODIUM 575mg; CALC 112mg

RECIPE BENEFITS: low-fat; high-fiber

CHOICE INGREDIENT: Look for small, heavy, white fennel bulbs that are firm and free of cracks. The stalks should be crisp with feathery, bright green fronds. Store fennel bulbs in a perforated plastic bag in the refrigerator for up to five days.

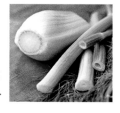

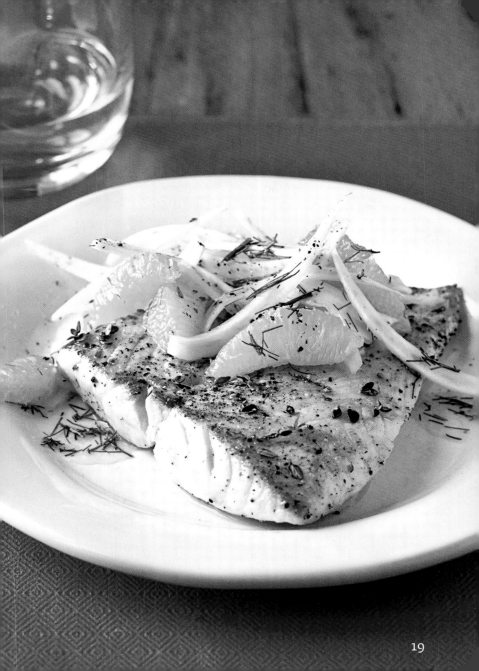

19

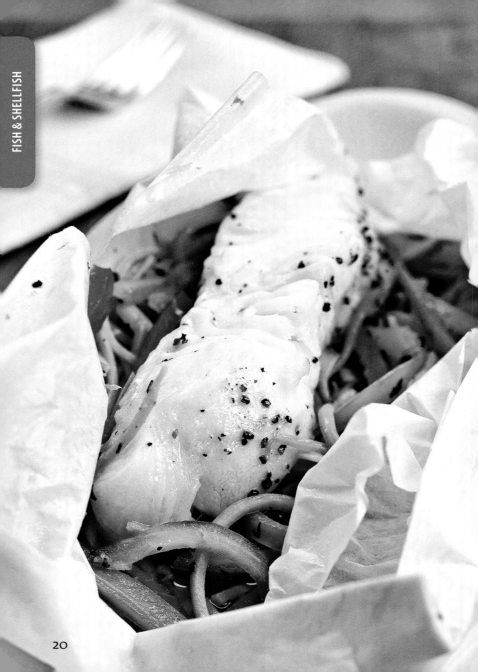

Gulf Fish en Papillote

En papillote is the French term for food baked in a parchment paper packet; it's a favorite way of preparing fish in New Orleans. This recipe easily doubles to serve four.

1 cup matchstick-cut carrots	¼ teaspoon salt, divided
1 cup vertically sliced red onion	¼ teaspoon freshly ground black pepper, divided
¾ cup (2-inch) julienne-cut celery	
½ cup red bell pepper strips	2 (6-ounce) sea bass fillets
1 teaspoon chopped fresh chervil	2 teaspoons butter, divided
1 teaspoon chopped fresh tarragon	¼ cup dry white wine, divided

1. Preheat oven to 350°.

2. Combine first 6 ingredients, ⅛ teaspoon salt, and ⅛ teaspoon pepper in a medium bowl.

3. Sprinkle fish evenly with remaining ⅛ teaspoon salt and ⅛ teaspoon pepper. Cut 2 (15-inch) squares of parchment paper. Fold each square in half, and open each. Place half of vegetable mixture near each fold. Top each serving with 1 fillet, 1 teaspoon butter, and 2 tablespoons wine. Fold paper; seal edges with narrow folds. Place packets on a jelly-roll pan. Bake at 350° for 18 minutes or until parchment is puffy. Place on plates, and cut open. Serve immediately. **YIELD:** 2 servings (serving size: 1 fillet and about 1½ cups vegetable mixture).

CALORIES 264; FAT 7.6g (sat 3.3g, mono 1.7g, poly 1.6g); PROTEIN 33.2g; CARB 15.4g; FIBER 3.8g; CHOL 80mg; IRON 1.2mg; SODIUM 518mg; CALC 77mg

RECIPE BENEFIT: low-fat

QUICK&EASY

Maple Grilled Salmon

The sweet-sour marinade is cooked down to a syrupy glaze that's brushed on the fish as it cooks. The citrus and maple flavors would also be tasty with pork. Garnish fillets with orange slices, if desired.

1/4 cup rice wine vinegar
3 tablespoons maple syrup
2 tablespoons fresh orange juice
4 (6-ounce) salmon fillets, skinned

Cooking spray
1/4 teaspoon salt
1/4 teaspoon freshly ground black pepper

1. Combine first 3 ingredients in a large zip-top plastic bag; add fish. Seal and marinate in refrigerator 3 hours.
2. Preheat grill or grill pan to medium-high heat.
3. Remove fish from bag, reserving marinade. Pour marinade into a small saucepan, and bring to a boil. Cook until reduced to 2 tablespoons (about 5 minutes).
4. Place fish on grill rack or pan coated with cooking spray; grill 4 minutes on each side or until fish flakes easily when tested with a fork or until desired degree of doneness, basting occasionally with marinade. Remove fish from grill; sprinkle with salt and pepper. **YIELD:** 4 servings (serving size: 1 fillet).

CALORIES 270; FAT 10.6g (sat 2.5g, mono 4.6g, poly 2.5g); PROTEIN 31.1g; CARB 11g; FIBER 0.1g; CHOL 80mg; IRON 0.7mg; SODIUM 216mg; CALC 27mg

RECIPE BENEFITS: low-fat; high-fiber

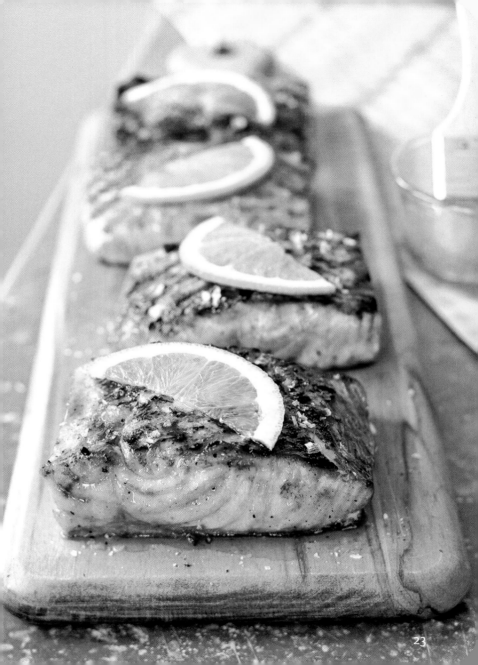

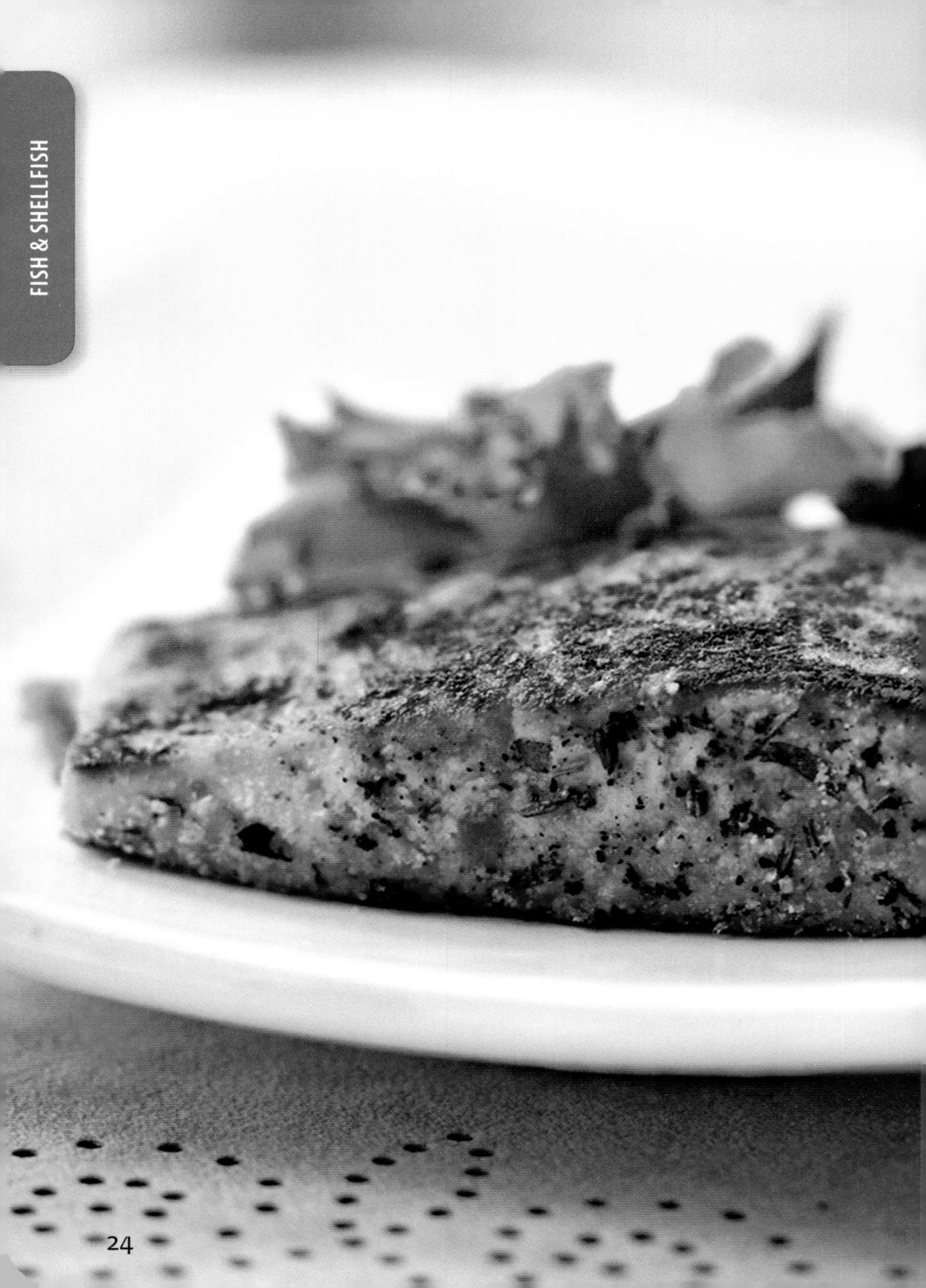

Herb-Crusted Salmon with Mixed Greens Salad

Chopped fresh herbs dress up salmon fillets. The homemade vinaigrette brightens salad greens while keeping calories and fat in check. Serve salmon with lemon wedges.

- ½ cup dry breadcrumbs
- 2 teaspoons chopped fresh oregano
- 2 teaspoons chopped fresh rosemary
- 2 teaspoons chopped fresh flat-leaf parsley
- 1½ teaspoons grated lemon rind
- ½ teaspoon black pepper
- 2 garlic cloves, minced
- 4 (6-ounce) salmon fillets (about 1 inch thick), skinned
- Cooking spray
- ¼ teaspoon kosher salt
- 1 tablespoon fresh lemon juice
- 1 tablespoon extra-virgin olive oil
- 1 teaspoon Dijon mustard
- ¼ teaspoon kosher salt
- ¼ teaspoon black pepper
- 4 cups mixed salad greens

1. Combine first 7 ingredients in a shallow dish or pie plate. Lightly coat both sides of fillets with cooking spray, and sprinkle evenly with ¼ teaspoon salt. Dredge both sides of fillets in breadcrumb mixture.

2. Heat a large nonstick skillet over medium-high heat. Coat pan with cooking spray. Add fillets to pan; cook 3 minutes. Reduce heat to medium; carefully turn fillets over. Cook 4 minutes or until fish flakes easily when tested with a fork or until desired degree of doneness.

3. To prepare salad, combine juice, oil, mustard, ¼ teaspoon salt, and ¼ teaspoon pepper in a large bowl. Add mixed greens; toss gently to coat. YIELD: 4 servings (serving size: 1 fillet and ⅔ cup salad).

CALORIES 256; FAT 9.5g (sat 2g, mono 4.6g, poly 2.2g); PROTEIN 32.1g; CARB 9g; FIBER 1.8g; CHOL 70mg; IRON 2mg; SODIUM 399mg; CALC 110mg

RECIPE BENEFITS: healthy fats; low-sodium

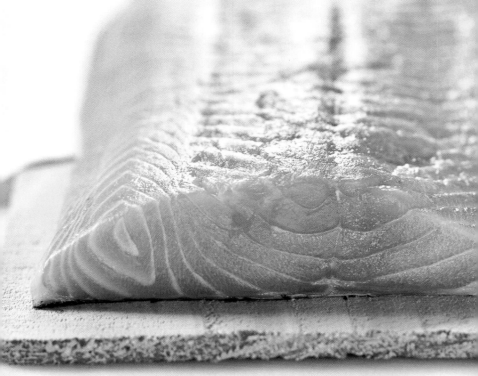

Salmon Nutrition

HOW DIFFERENT VARIETIES OF SALMON COMPARE

The American Heart Association recommends eating salmon or other fatty fish, such as mackerel or tuna, twice each week for the heart-protective benefits associated with omega-3 fatty acids found in their fish oils. The marketplace obliges, offering wild-caught, farm-raised, canned, and smoked salmon. But according to USDA figures, there are nutritional differences, depending on the source and methods of preparation.

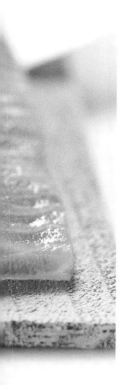

FARM-RAISED: Farmed salmon generally contains more calories, more fat and, consequently, more omega-3 fatty acids than wild fish (2.147 grams versus 1.059). Farm-raised flavors tend to be milder.

WILD-CAUGHT: Aficionados favor sea-running salmon for its more assertive flavor, particularly chinook and coho. And fresh salmon, both wild and farmed, deliver more protein than processed varieties (for example, 23 grams for wild coho versus 18 for smoked). Ask your fishmonger which is freshest, as nutritional values degrade over time.

CANNED: The most commonly canned species are pink and sockeye salmon. Between the two, the cheaper pink has the edge in higher omega-3 values (1.65 grams versus 1.15 grams), though the stronger-tasting, firmer-textured, red-hued sockeye tends to win flavor comparisons. Soft fish bones found in canned varieties deliver high calcium levels, giving them a strong nutritional edge. Salt used to preserve the fish contributes to moderate sodium levels, though.

SMOKED: Smoking preserves salmon by exposing it to high heat, resulting in smoky, flaky fish. To get the smooth texture associated with lox, salmon is dunked in salt brine and then "cold smoked" at a lower temperature for a longer time. Both smoking processes degrade protein, fat, and omega-3 values from fresh fish and increase salt content significantly. Ordinary smoked salmon has 784 grams of sodium, and a typical serving of lox contains a whopping 2,000 grams, which is almost equal to the Recommended Daily Intake.

(Values reflect 3.5-ounce servings.)

Tuna with Avocado Green Goddess Aïoli

The aïoli features heart-healthy avocado, which contributes vitamin E to this dish. But the real nutritional standout is the tuna, which is rich in niacin.

$1/4$ cup fat-free sour cream

2 tablespoons chopped fresh cilantro

1 tablespoon chopped fresh basil leaves

1 tablespoon chopped fresh flat-leaf parsley

6 tablespoons chopped ripe peeled avocado

2 tablespoons fat-free mayonnaise

1 teaspoon fresh lemon juice

$1/4$ teaspoon salt

1 garlic clove, chopped

$3/4$ teaspoon ground coriander

$1/2$ teaspoon salt

$1/2$ teaspoon ground cumin

$1/2$ teaspoon garlic powder

$1/4$ teaspoon chili powder

$1/8$ teaspoon freshly ground black pepper

4 (6-ounce) tuna steaks (about 1 inch thick)

Cooking spray

1. Place first 9 ingredients in a blender; process until smooth.

2. Combine coriander and next 5 ingredients in a small bowl; sprinkle spice mixture evenly over tuna.

3. Heat a grill pan over medium-high heat. Coat pan with cooking spray. Add tuna; cook 2 minutes on each side or until medium-rare or desired degree of doneness. Serve with aïoli. YIELD: 4 servings (serving size: 1 tuna steak and about $2^1/2$ tablespoons aïoli).

CALORIES 234; FAT 6.1g (sat 1.8g, mono 2.6g, poly 1.2g); PROTEIN 39g; CARB 6.1g; FIBER 1.3g; CHOL 82mg; IRON 2.4mg; SODIUM 581mg; CALC 82mg

RECIPE BENEFIT: healthy fats

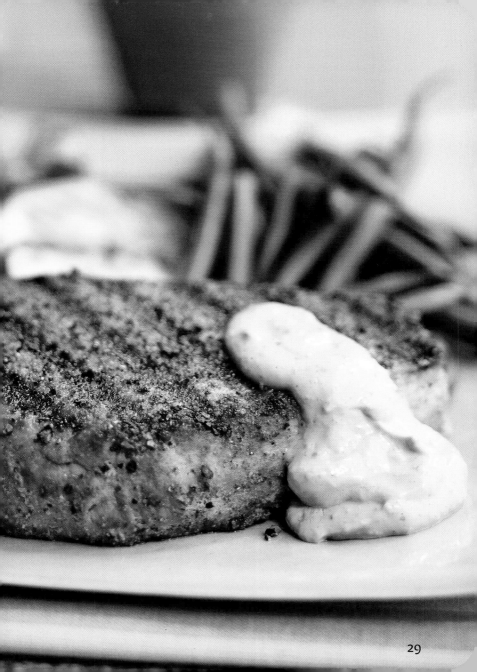

Grilled Tuna with Chipotle Ponzu and Avocado Salsa

Here is a great example of how bold Asian and Latin flavors work well together. Orange and lime juice substitute for rice vinegar, the acidic ingredient typically used in a Japanese ponzu dipping sauce. It gets a kick from the hot, smoky chipotle chiles. You can also try the ponzu with chicken.

$1/2$ cup orange juice	$1/2$ cup diced plum tomato
$1/2$ cup lime juice	$1/2$ cup diced peeled avocado
$1/4$ cup grated onion	$1/4$ cup chopped fresh cilantro
$1/4$ cup low-sodium soy sauce	4 (6-ounce) tuna steaks
1 tablespoon chopped peeled fresh ginger	$1/4$ teaspoon salt
	Cooking spray
$1^1/2$ chipotle chiles in adobo sauce	2 cups hot cooked medium-grain rice
$3/4$ cup diced English cucumber	

1. Place $1/2$ cup orange juice and next 5 ingredients in a blender, and process until smooth.

2. Combine diced cucumber, tomato, avocado, and cilantro in a small bowl.

3. Sprinkle fish with salt. Heat a large nonstick grill pan over medium-high heat. Coat pan with cooking spray. Add fish; cook 3 minutes on each side or until desired degree of doneness. Cut each tuna steak diagonally across the grain into thin slices. Arrange sliced tuna over rice; top with salsa, and drizzle with ponzu. **YIELD:** 4 servings (serving size: 1 tuna steak, $1/2$ cup rice, $1/2$ cup salsa, and about $1/3$ cup ponzu).

CALORIES 447; FAT 12.6g (sat 2.8g, mono 5.2g, poly 3.1g); PROTEIN 44g; CARB 37.8g; FIBER 2.5g; CHOL 64mg; IRON 3.9mg; SODIUM 606mg; CALC 34mg

RECIPE BENEFIT: healthy fats

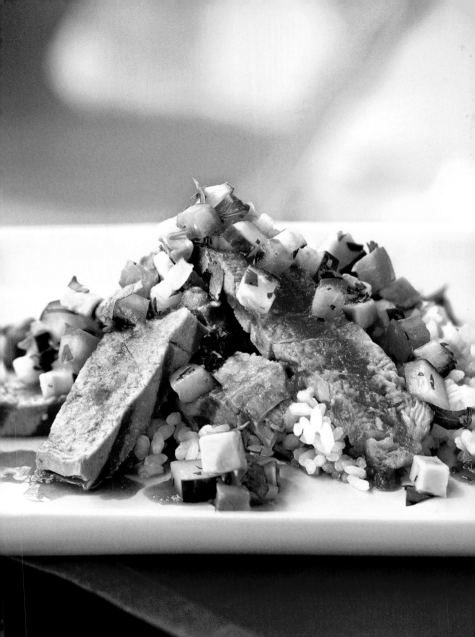

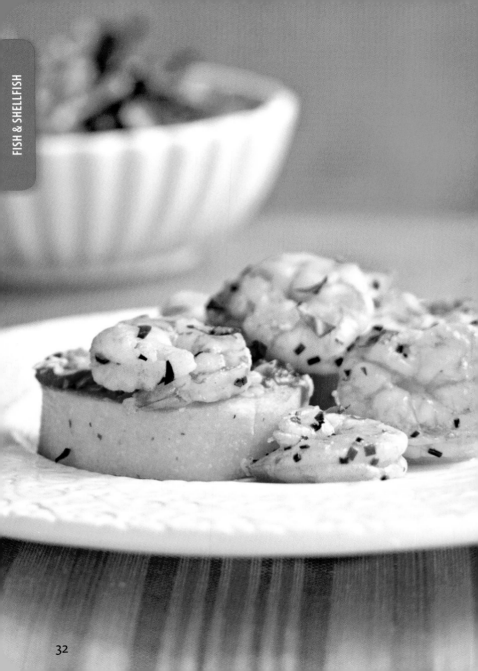

Smoky Shrimp and Parmesan-Polenta Cakes

Smoked paprika, available in supermarkets, is nice to spice up sour cream, eggs, or rice. Its pungency offsets the shrimp's sweetness. Serve with bagged prewashed salad greens splashed with vinaigrette.

1 tablespoon olive oil
1 pound peeled and deveined medium shrimp
¼ cup dry white wine
1 tablespoon chopped fresh chives
1 tablespoon fresh lemon juice
¼ teaspoon Spanish smoked paprika

1 17-ounce tube polenta, cut into 8 (½-inch) slices
Cooking spray
8 teaspoons marinara sauce
8 teaspoons grated fresh Parmesan cheese
1 tablespoon chopped fresh flat-leaf parsley

1. Preheat broiler.

2. Heat oil in a large skillet over medium-high heat. Add shrimp to pan; sauté 3 minutes or until done, stirring frequently. Remove from heat; stir in wine, chives, juice, and paprika, tossing to coat. Keep warm.

3. Place polenta slices on a baking sheet coated with cooking spray. Top each slice with 1 teaspoon sauce and 1 teaspoon cheese; broil 3 minutes or until cheese melts. Place 2 polenta slices on each of 4 plates; top each serving evenly with shrimp mixture. Sprinkle with parsley. **YIELD:** 4 servings.

CALORIES 231; FAT 5.4g (sat 1.3g, mono 2.9g, poly 0.8g); PROTEIN 21.7g; CARB 18.8g; FIBER 2.4g; CHOL 171mg; IRON 3.7mg; SODIUM 386mg; CALC 75mg

RECIPE BENEFITS: low-fat; low-sodium

Shrimp

BESIDES THEIR SUCCULENT FLAVOR, the culinary versatility and largely year-round availability of shrimp are likely what makes them so popular. And despite the fact that shrimp contain more cholesterol than some other types of seafood, the total fat and saturated fat (the real culprit in heart disease) content is very low. So we think it's fine to include shrimp in a heart-healthy diet.

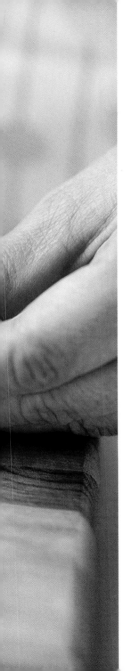

HOW MUCH SHRIMP TO BUY: To save prep time, instead of peeling and deveining your own shrimp, you can buy peeled and deveined raw shrimp at the seafood counter of most supermarkets. The chart below shows how much peeled and deveined shrimp to buy when the recipe calls for unpeeled shrimp.

RAW SHRIMP UNPEELED		RAW SHRIMP PEELED & DEVEINED
⅔ pound	=	½ pound
1 pound	=	¾ pound
1⅓ pounds	=	1 pound
2 pounds	=	1½ pounds
2⅔ pounds	=	2 pounds
4 pounds	=	3 pounds

HOW TO STORE SHRIMP: Fresh uncooked shrimp is very perishable, so use it within two days of purchase. After bringing it home, rinse thoroughly under cold running water, and pat dry with paper towels. Cover shrimp loosely with wax paper so that air can circulate around it; store in the coolest part of the refrigerator, preferably on a bed of ice. Shrimp can be frozen, but they lose some of their texture after thawing. When you want to use frozen shrimp, just thaw them in a bowl or sink filled with tap water.

HOW TO PEEL AND DEVEIN SHRIMP: Except for the largest shrimp, there's neither danger nor distaste in leaving the thin black line (vein) right where it is.

1. Peel the shell off the shrimp.
2. Cut a shallow slit along the back using a sharp paring knife.
3. Remove the dark vein using a sharp knife or deveining tool.
4. Rinse under cold water, and drain.

Sesame Shrimp Salad

1 tablespoon sugar
3 tablespoons fresh lime juice, divided
1 tablespoon water
1 garlic clove, minced
2 teaspoons chili garlic sauce (such as Lee Kum Kee), divided
1½ teaspoons fish sauce
½ teaspoon salt, divided
1 tablespoon orange marmalade
2 teaspoons dark sesame oil, divided
24 large shrimp, peeled and deveined (about 1 pound)
5 cups shredded napa (Chinese) cabbage
1½ cups trimmed watercress leaves
1½ cups shredded carrot
⅓ cup chopped fresh cilantro
⅓ cup chopped fresh mint
2 tablespoons toasted sesame seeds

1. Combine sugar, 2 tablespoons juice, 1 tablespoon water, and garlic in a small microwave-safe bowl; cover with plastic wrap. Microwave at HIGH 40 seconds or until sugar dissolves. Cool. Stir in 1 teaspoon chili garlic sauce, fish sauce, and ¼ teaspoon salt.

2. Combine remaining 1 tablespoon juice, remaining 1 teaspoon chili garlic sauce, remaining ¼ teaspoon salt, marmalade, and 1 teaspoon oil in a large bowl, stirring with a whisk. Add shrimp to bowl; toss to coat. Marinate shrimp in refrigerator 15 minutes, tossing occasionally. Remove shrimp from bowl, reserving marinade. Thread 3 shrimp onto each of 8 (8-inch) wooden skewers.

3. Heat 1 teaspoon oil in a large nonstick skillet over medium-high heat. Add skewers and reserved marinade to pan; cook 3½ minutes or until shrimp is done and glazed, turning once.

4. Combine cabbage and remaining ingredients in a large bowl. Drizzle fish sauce mixture over cabbage; toss well. **YIELD:** 4 servings (serving size: 2 skewers and 2 cups cabbage mixture).

CALORIES 239; FAT 7.3g (sat 1.2g, mono 2.4g, poly 3g); PROTEIN 26.3g; CARB 17.9g; FIBER 3.4g; CHOL 172mg; IRON 3.4mg; SODIUM 726mg; CALC 179mg

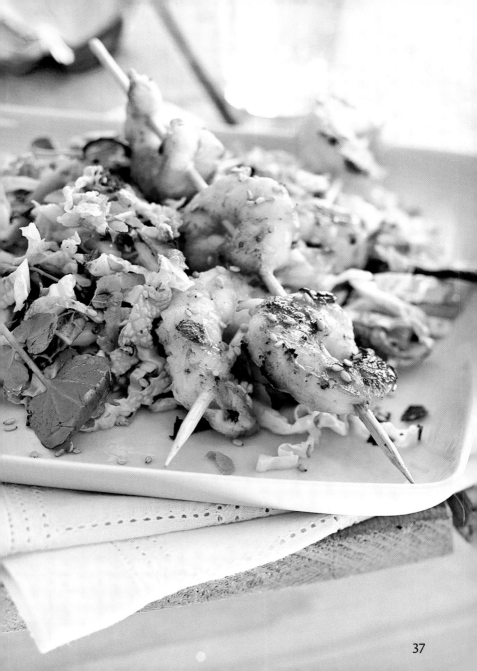

take two:

Shrimp vs.
Scallops

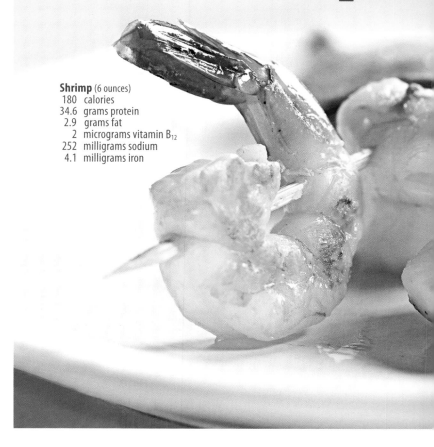

Shrimp (6 ounces)
- 180 calories
- 34.6 grams protein
- 2.9 grams fat
- 2 micrograms vitamin B_{12}
- 252 milligrams sodium
- 4.1 milligrams iron

Shrimp and scallops are great for a quick meal any night of the week.

Either can be quickly sautéed and then added to salads and pastas or served solo as an entrée or appetizer. Similar portions offer filling protein with relatively few calories and little fat. And each contains comparable sodium profiles—about 10 percent of your daily allotment—and almost a day's worth of vitamin B12, a nutrient that helps support metabolism. However, a serving of shrimp yields about eight times as much iron (nearly one-fourth of a woman's daily needs).

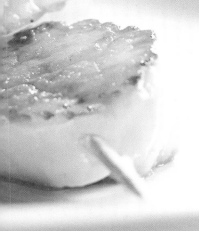

Scallops (6 ounces)
- 150 calories
- 28.5 grams protein
- 1.3 grams fat
- 2.6 micrograms vitamin B_{12}
- 274 milligrams sodium
- 0.5 milligrams iron

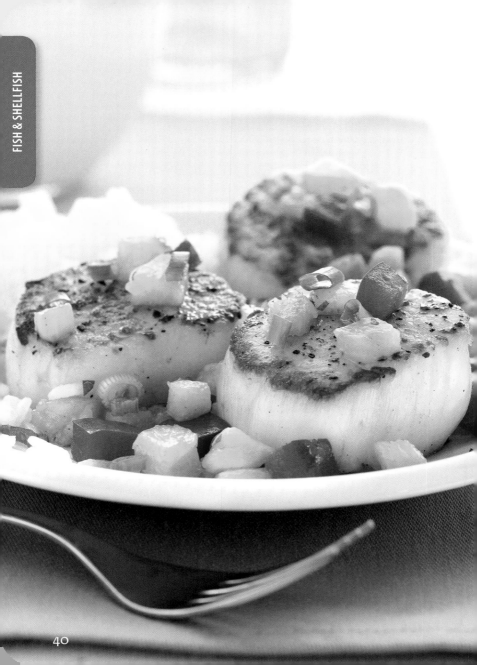

Seared Scallops with Warm Fruit Salsa

A hot skillet is key to a deep golden sear on the scallops. Prepare the salsa in the same skillet as the scallops for an easy one-pan cleanup. Jasmine rice rounds out the meal.

12 large sea scallops (about 1¼ pounds)
Cooking spray
¼ teaspoon freshly ground black pepper
⅛ teaspoon salt
2 teaspoons olive oil
1 garlic clove, minced
2 cups diced pineapple
1¼ cups chopped red bell pepper
¼ cup green tea with mango (such as Snapple)
2 teaspoons low-sodium soy sauce
1 tablespoon chopped fresh mint
4 teaspoons sliced green onions

1. Pat scallops dry with paper towels. Heat a large nonstick skillet over medium-high heat. Coat pan with cooking spray. Sprinkle scallops evenly with pepper and salt. Add scallops to pan; cook 3 minutes on each side or until done. Remove scallops from pan; keep warm.
2. Heat oil in a large nonstick skillet over medium-high heat. Add garlic; sauté 1 minute. Stir in pineapple and next 3 ingredients, scraping pan to loosen browned bits; cook 3 minutes. Stir in mint.
3. Discard any accumulated juices from scallops; top evenly with salsa and onions. Serve immediately. **YIELD:** 4 servings (serving size: 3 scallops and about ⅔ cup salsa).

CALORIES 202; FAT 4g (sat 0.5g, mono 1.7g, poly 0.8g); PROTEIN 24.9g; CARB 17.7g; FIBER 2.2g; CHOL 47mg; IRON 1mg; SODIUM 394mg; CALC 52mg

RECIPE BENEFITS: low-fat; low-sodium

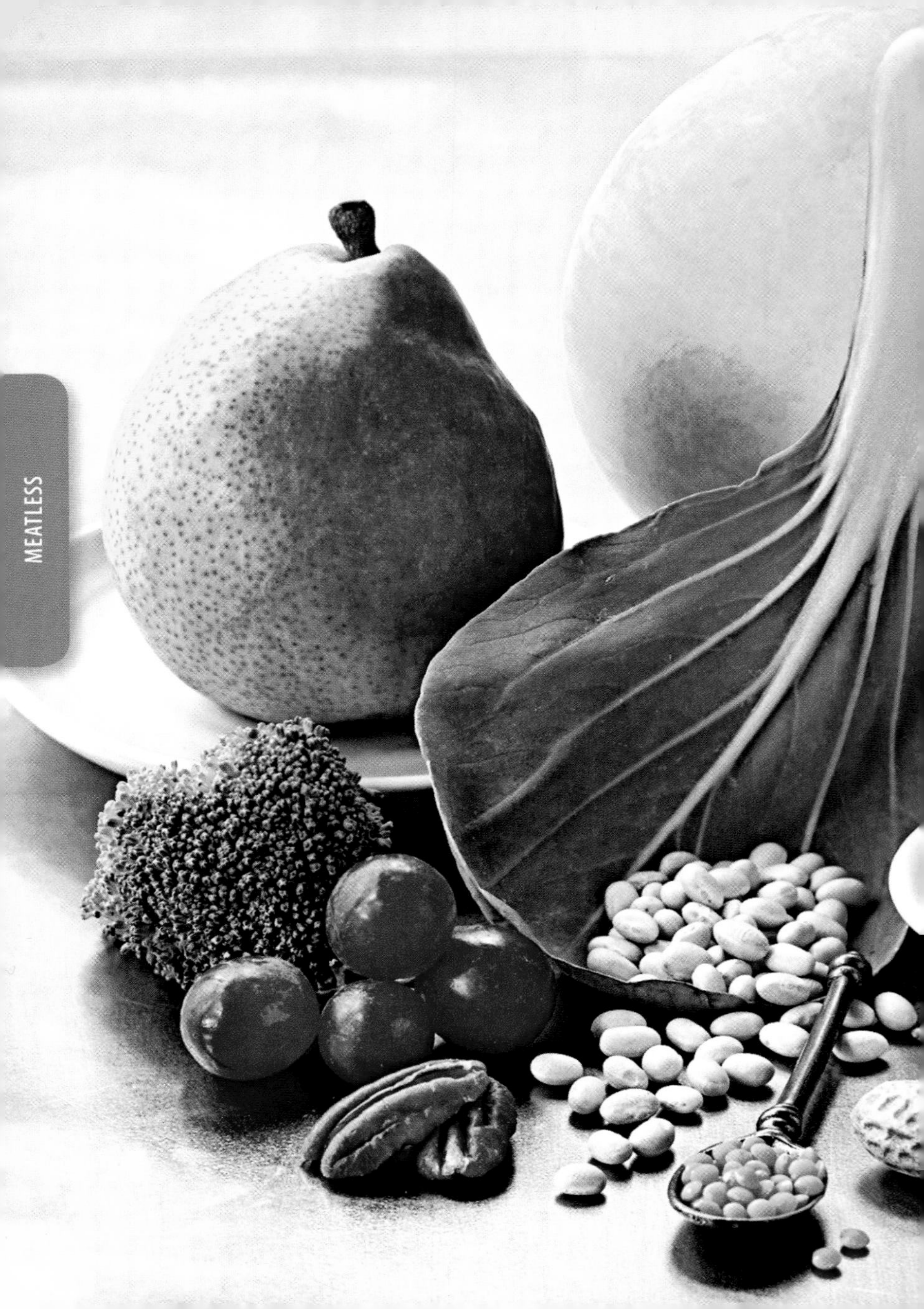

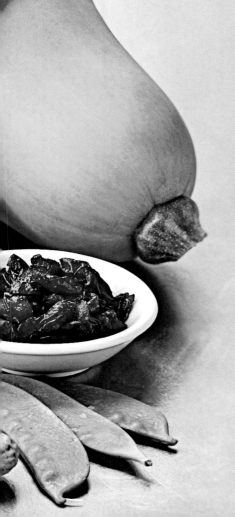

Meatless

Flexitarianism

A flexible take on vegetarianism, this approach involves a primarily plant-based diet supplemented with occasional protein.

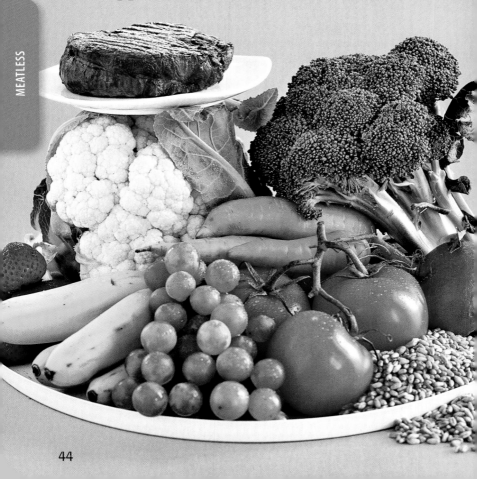

Like vegetarians, "flexitarians" eat a primarily plant-based diet composed of grains, vegetables, and fruits, but they occasionally obtain protein from lean meat, fish, poultry, or dairy. A quarter of Americans fit the description, consuming meatless meals at least four days a week, according to the American Dietetic Association (ADA).

Why it's here to stay:

Flexitarianism is exactly what dietitians, nutritional researchers, and public health advocates have been recommending for years—a varied diet that's low in saturated fat and high in fiber. Because the emphasis is on produce rather than protein, flexitarians are more likely than most Americans to meet the recommended daily intake of fruits and vegetables and the vitamins and minerals they contain.

What it means for you:

Studies show that people who follow this approach to eating generally weigh less and have lower rates of hypertension, heart disease, diabetes, and prostate and colon cancer. In one large study from Tulane University in New Orleans, researchers tracked the eating habits of more than 9,600 people over a 19-year period and found those who consumed fruits and vegetables at least three times daily lowered their risk of stroke by 42 percent and their risk of cardiovascular disease by 27 percent.

Red Lentil–Rice Cakes with Tomato Salsa

3 cups finely chopped plum tomato (about 6 tomatoes)
1/4 cup chopped fresh basil
1 tablespoon balsamic vinegar
2 teaspoons capers
1/4 teaspoon salt
5 cups water, divided
1 cup dried small red lentils
1/2 cup uncooked basmati rice
2 tablespoons olive oil, divided
1/2 cup finely chopped red bell pepper

1/2 cup finely chopped red onion
1/2 teaspoon fennel seeds, crushed
2 garlic cloves, minced
3/4 cup (3 ounces) shredded part-skim mozzarella cheese
1/4 cup dry breadcrumbs
1 tablespoon chopped fresh basil
1 teaspoon salt
1/4 teaspoon freshly ground black pepper
2 large egg whites, lightly beaten

1. Combine first 5 ingredients. Bring 4 cups water and lentils to a boil in a saucepan. Reduce heat; simmer 20 minutes or until tender. Drain; rinse lentils, and place in a large bowl.

2. Combine 1 cup water and rice in pan; bring to a boil. Cover, reduce heat, and simmer 18 minutes or until liquid is absorbed. Cool 10 minutes. Add rice to lentils.

3. Heat 1 teaspoon oil in a large nonstick skillet over medium-high heat. Add bell pepper and next 3 ingredients to pan; sauté 2 minutes or until tender. Cool 10 minutes. Add to rice mixture. Add cheese and remaining ingredients; stir well. Let stand 10 minutes.

4. Wipe skillet clean. Heat 2 teaspoons oil in skillet over medium heat. Spoon half of rice mixture by 1/3-cupfuls into pan, spreading to form 6 (3-inch) circles. Cook 5 minutes or until browned. Turn cakes over; cook 5 minutes. Remove cakes from pan. Repeat procedure with remaining 1 tablespoon oil and remaining rice mixture. Serve with salsa. **YIELD:** 6 servings (serving size: 2 cakes and 1/2 cup salsa).

CALORIES 279; FAT 8.7g (sat 2.5g, mono 4.2g, poly 0.8g); PROTEIN 15.9g; CARB 35.8g; FIBER 6.6g; CHOL 8mg; IRON 2.8mg; SODIUM 660mg; CALC 142mg

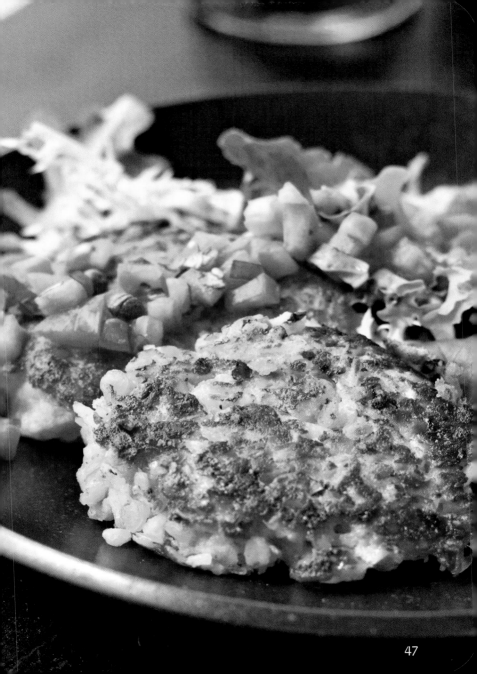

White Beans with Roasted Red Pepper and Pesto

2 cups loosely packed basil leaves
$^1/_2$ cup (2 ounces) grated fresh Parmesan cheese
2 tablespoons pine nuts, toasted
2 tablespoons water
2 tablespoons extra-virgin olive oil
1 garlic clove, crushed
$1^1/_4$ teaspoons salt, divided
$^3/_8$ teaspoon freshly ground black pepper, divided

1 pound dried Great Northern beans
10 cups water, divided
$1^1/_2$ cups coarsely chopped onion
1 tablespoon chopped fresh sage
1 tablespoon olive oil
2 garlic cloves, crushed
1 cup chopped bottled roasted red bell peppers
1 tablespoon balsamic vinegar

1. Place first 6 ingredients, $^1/_4$ teaspoon salt, and $^1/_8$ teaspoon black pepper in a food processor; process until smooth.

2. Sort and wash beans. Combine beans and 4 cups water in a 6-quart pressure cooker. Close lid securely; bring to high pressure over high heat. Adjust heat to medium or level needed to maintain high pressure, and cook 3 minutes. Remove from heat; place cooker under cold running water. Remove lid; drain beans.

3. Combine beans, 6 cups water, onion, and next 3 ingredients in cooker. Close lid securely; bring to high pressure over high heat. Adjust heat to medium or level needed to maintain high pressure; cook 12 minutes. Remove from heat; place cooker under cold running water. Remove lid; let stand 10 minutes. Drain in a colander over a bowl, reserving 1 cup liquid. Return bean mixture and reserved 1 cup liquid to cooker. Add 1 teaspoon salt, $^1/_4$ teaspoon black pepper, bell peppers, and vinegar. Stir well to combine. Top with pesto. **YIELD:** 8 servings (serving size: about $^3/_4$ cup bean mixture and 2 tablespoons pesto).

CALORIES 292; FAT 8g (sat 2.1g, mono 4.1g, poly 1.2g); PROTEIN 16.3g; CARB 40.5g; FIBER 12.7g; CHOL 5mg; IRON 3.9mg; SODIUM 542mg; CALC 212mg

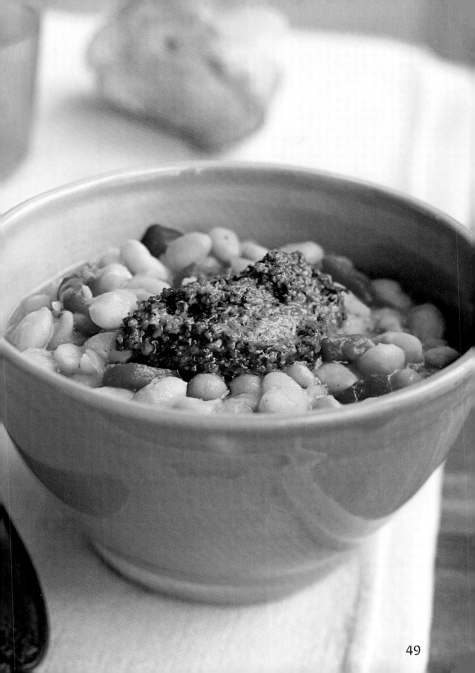

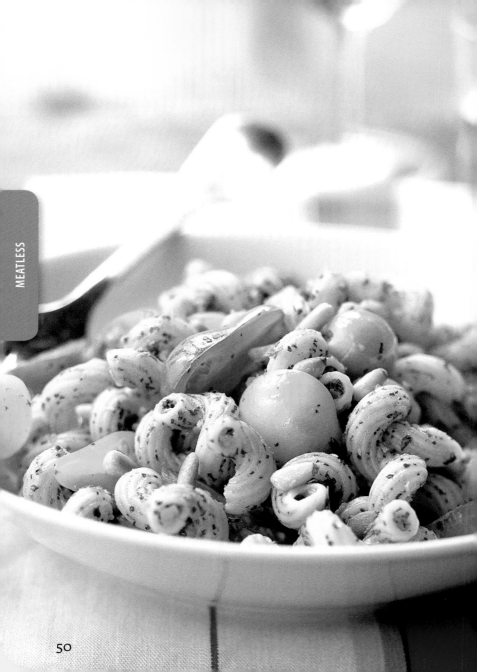

Cavatappi with Arugula Pesto and Grape Tomatoes

Peppery arugula complements the sweetness of ripe tomatoes. Use multicolored tomatoes, if available, for even better flavor. Substitute fusilli for cavatappi, if desired. Serve immediately.

5 cups trimmed arugula
1/2 cup (2 ounces) grated fresh Parmesan cheese
1/4 cup pine nuts, toasted
1 tablespoon lemon juice
3/4 teaspoon salt
1/4 teaspoon freshly ground black pepper
1 garlic clove, minced

1/3 cup water
2 tablespoons extra-virgin olive oil
1 pound uncooked cavatappi
2 cups red and yellow grape tomatoes, halved (about 3/4 pound)
2 tablespoons pine nuts, toasted

1. To prepare pesto, place first 7 ingredients in a food processor; process until finely minced. With processor on, slowly pour 1/3 cup water and oil through food chute; process until well blended.
2. Cook pasta according to package directions, omitting salt and fat. Drain. Combine pesto, pasta, and tomatoes in a large bowl; toss well. Sprinkle pine nuts over pasta. Serve immediately. **YIELD:** 6 servings (serving size: 1 1/3 cups pasta and 1 teaspoon nuts).

CALORIES 425; FAT 13.7g (sat 2.8g, mono 6.3g, poly 3.7g); PROTEIN 14.6g; CARB 61.5g; FIBER 3.2g; CHOL 6mg; IRON 2.1mg; SODIUM 412mg; CALC 135mg

RECIPE BENEFIT: low-sodium

QUICK&EASY

Pasta with Zucchini and Toasted Almonds

For a superfast and delicious meal in minutes, pair the flavorful pasta with store-bought breadsticks or a lower-sodium option of fresh, prechopped melon.

2 cups cherry tomatoes, halved
2 tablespoons minced shallots
1 teaspoon minced fresh thyme
2 teaspoons fresh lemon juice
3/4 teaspoon kosher salt
1/2 teaspoon freshly ground black pepper
1/4 teaspoon sugar
5 teaspoons extra-virgin olive oil, divided
1 (9-ounce) package refrigerated linguine

1 1/2 teaspoons bottled minced garlic
3 cups chopped zucchini (about 1 pound)
3/4 cup fat-free, less-sodium chicken broth
3 tablespoons chopped fresh mint, divided
1/3 cup (1 1/2 ounces) grated fresh pecorino Romano cheese
3 tablespoons sliced almonds, toasted

1. Combine first 7 ingredients in a medium bowl. Add 2 teaspoons oil, tossing to coat.

2. Cook pasta according to package directions, omitting salt and fat. Drain well.

3. Heat a large nonstick skillet over medium-high heat. Add remaining 1 tablespoon oil to pan, swirling to coat. Add garlic to pan; sauté 30 seconds. Add zucchini; sauté 3 minutes or until crisp-tender. Add broth; bring to a simmer. Stir in pasta and 1 1/2 tablespoons mint; toss well. Remove from heat; stir in tomato mixture. Place 1 1/2 cups pasta mixture in each of 4 bowls; top evenly with remaining 1 1/2 tablespoons mint. Sprinkle each serving with 4 teaspoons cheese and 2 teaspoons almonds. YIELD: 4 servings.

CALORIES 344; FAT 12.7g (sat 3.1g, mono 6.6g, poly 2g); PROTEIN 14g; CARB 45.5g; FIBER 5.3g; CHOL 58mg; IRON 3.4mg; SODIUM 601mg; CALC 163mg

RECIPE BENEFIT: high-fiber

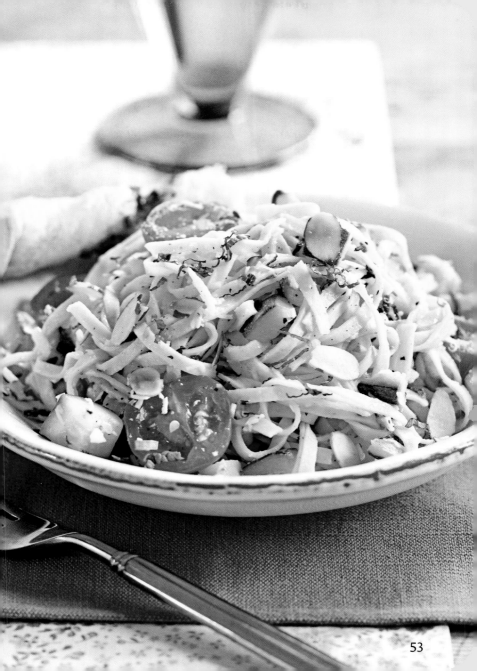

Sautéed Vegetables and Spicy Tofu

Thanks to a package of seasoned tofu, this easy stir-fry comes together in a snap. This dish is delicious served alone, but for heartier fare, serve it on top of rice noodles.

1 **(16-ounce) package spicy tofu, drained**
2 **tablespoons olive oil, divided**
2 **tablespoons fresh lemon juice**
$\frac{1}{2}$ **teaspoon salt**
$\frac{1}{4}$ **teaspoon crushed red pepper**

2 **large garlic cloves, pressed**
1 **large zucchini, halved lengthwise and cut crosswise into thin slices**
1 **cup thinly sliced red bell pepper**
Lemon wedges (optional)

1. Place tofu on several layers of heavy-duty paper towels. Cover tofu with additional paper towels; gently press out moisture. Cut tofu into $\frac{1}{2}$-inch cubes.

2. Combine 1 tablespoon oil and next 4 ingredients in a medium bowl. Set aside.

3. Heat remaining 1 tablespoon oil in a large nonstick skillet over medium-high heat. Add tofu, zucchini, and bell pepper; stir-fry 8 to 10 minutes or until tofu is browned and vegetables are crisp-tender. Add oil mixture; cook 1 minute, stirring gently. Serve with lemon wedges, if desired. **YIELD:** 4 servings (serving size: 1 cup).

CALORIES 196; FAT 13.7g (sat 2.3g, mono 5g, poly 5g); PROTEIN 15g; CARB 7.9g; FIBER 3.2g; CHOL 0mg; IRON 3mg; SODIUM 302mg; CALC 154mg

RECIPE BENEFIT: healthy fats

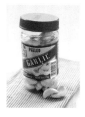

QUICK TIP: Reduce meal prep time by using jarred, pre-peeled garlic cloves instead of peeling them yourself. Look for them in the refrigerated produce section at your supermarket.

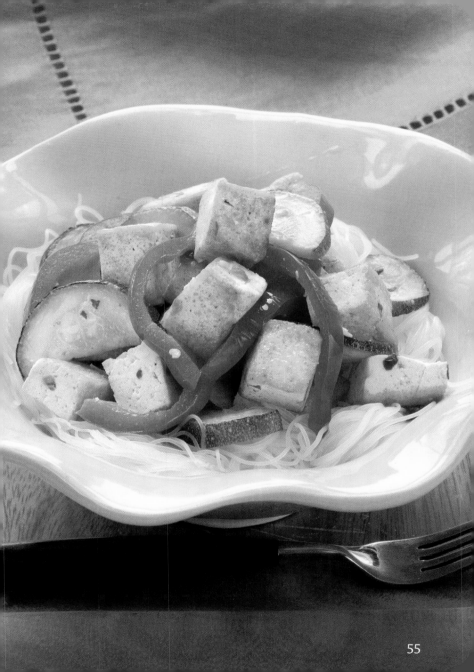

Summer Squash Pizza

You can use all zucchini or yellow squash for this grilled pie. Serve one slice as an appetizer or two with a salad for a simple supper.

1 teaspoon olive oil
1 teaspoon balsamic vinegar
$^1/_8$ teaspoon salt
$^1/_8$ teaspoon freshly ground black pepper
1 medium zucchini, cut lengthwise into ($^1/_4$-inch-thick) slices
1 medium yellow squash, cut lengthwise into ($^1/_4$-inch-thick) slices
Cooking spray

1 (12-inch) packaged pizza crust (such as Mama Mary's)
2 plum tomatoes, cut into ($^1/_8$-inch-thick) slices
$^1/_4$ cup (1 ounce) finely grated pecorino Romano cheese
2 tablespoons thinly sliced fresh basil
$^1/_2$ teaspoon finely chopped fresh oregano

1. Prepare grill.

2. Combine oil, vinegar, salt, pepper, zucchini slices, and yellow squash slices in a large bowl, tossing gently to coat. Place squash mixture on grill rack coated with cooking spray; grill 2 minutes on each side or until tender.

3. Reduce grill temperature to medium.

4. Lightly coat pizza crust with cooking spray; grill 1 minute on each side or until lightly toasted. Arrange zucchini and squash over crust. Arrange tomatoes over squash; sprinkle with pecorino Romano cheese. Grill 5 minutes or until thoroughly heated. Remove from grill; sprinkle with basil and oregano.

YIELD: 8 servings (serving size: 1 slice).

CALORIES 165; FAT 6.1g (sat 1.5g, mono 0.7g, poly 0.1g); PROTEIN 5.6g; CARB 23.5g; FIBER 1.5g; CHOL 4mg; IRON 1.6mg; SODIUM 225mg; CALC 92mg

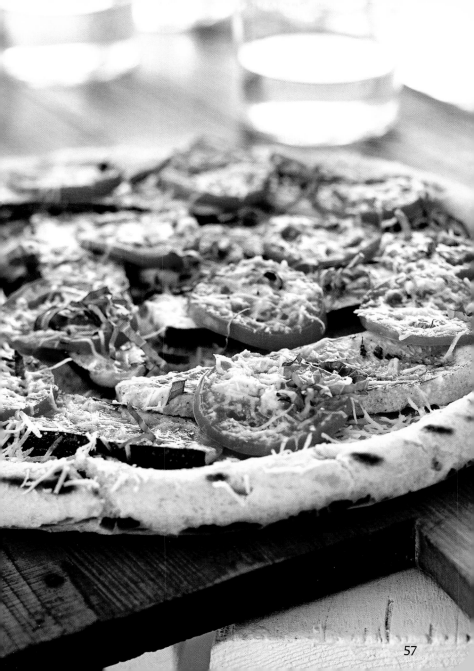

Black Lentil and Couscous Salad

This zesty side is modeled after tabbouleh, the Middle Eastern salad of bulgur wheat, tomatoes, cucumbers, herbs, lemon juice, and olive oil. Here, we use couscous instead of bulgur and add black lentils for color and texture. Serve chilled or at room temperature.

$1/2$ cup dried black lentils
5 cups water, divided
$3/4$ cup uncooked couscous
$3/4$ teaspoon salt, divided
1 cup cherry tomatoes, quartered
$1/3$ cup golden raisins
$1/3$ cup finely chopped red onion

$1/3$ cup finely chopped cucumber
$1/4$ cup chopped fresh parsley
3 tablespoons chopped fresh mint
1 teaspoon grated lemon rind
3 tablespoons fresh lemon juice
2 tablespoons extra-virgin olive oil

1. Rinse lentils with cold water; drain. Place lentils and 4 cups water in a large saucepan; bring to a boil. Reduce heat, and simmer 20 minutes or until tender. Drain and rinse with cold water; drain.

2. Bring remaining 1 cup water to a boil in a medium saucepan; gradually stir in couscous and $1/4$ teaspoon salt. Remove from heat; cover and let stand 5 minutes. Fluff with a fork. Combine lentils, couscous, remaining $1/2$ teaspoon salt, tomatoes, and remaining ingredients in a large bowl. **YIELD:** 6 servings (serving size: 1 cup).

CALORIES 175; FAT 4.8g (sat 0.7g, mono 3.3g, poly 0.6g); PROTEIN 4.5g; CARB 28.8g; FIBER 2.8g; CHOL 0mg; IRON 1mg; SODIUM 322mg; CALC 31mg

RECIPE BENEFIT: healthy fats

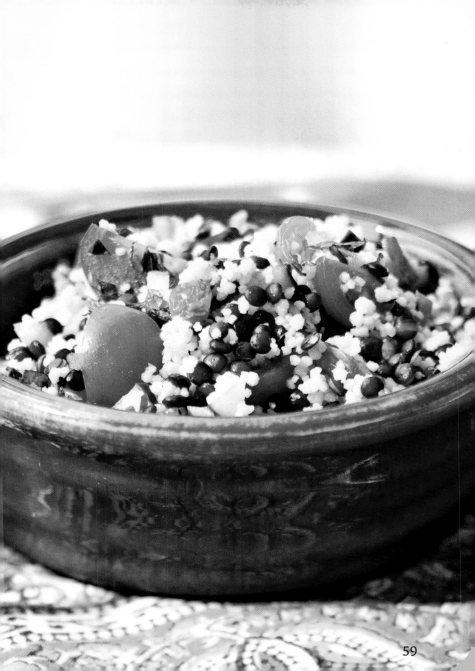

Bulgur Salad with Edamame and Cherry Tomatoes

The vitamin C from lemon juice aids iron absorption. Round out the meal with grilled chicken, lemony hummus, and toasted 100 percent whole-wheat pita wedges. Substitute fresh shelled fava beans for edamame, if you like. Fava beans also supply protein, fiber, and B vitamins.

1 cup uncooked bulgur
1 cup boiling water
1 cup frozen shelled edamame (green soybeans)
1 pound yellow and red cherry tomatoes, halved
1 cup finely chopped fresh flat-leaf parsley

$\frac{1}{3}$ cup finely chopped fresh mint
2 tablespoons chopped fresh dill
1 cup chopped green onions
$\frac{1}{4}$ cup fresh lemon juice
$\frac{1}{4}$ cup extra-virgin olive oil
1 teaspoon kosher salt
$\frac{1}{2}$ teaspoon freshly ground black pepper

1. Combine bulgur and 1 cup boiling water in a large bowl. Cover and let stand 1 hour or until bulgur is tender.

2. Cook edamame in boiling water 3 minutes or until crisp-tender. Drain. Add edamame, tomatoes, and remaining ingredients to bulgur; toss well. Let stand at room temperature 1 hour before serving. **YIELD:** 6 servings (serving size: $1\frac{1}{4}$ cups).

CALORIES 208; FAT 10.5g (sat 1.3g, mono 6.7g, poly 1.2g); PROTEIN 6.3g; CARB 25.4g; FIBER 7.1g; CHOL 0mg; IRON 2.2mg; SODIUM 332mg; CALC 59mg

RECIPE BENEFITS: healthy fats; high-fiber

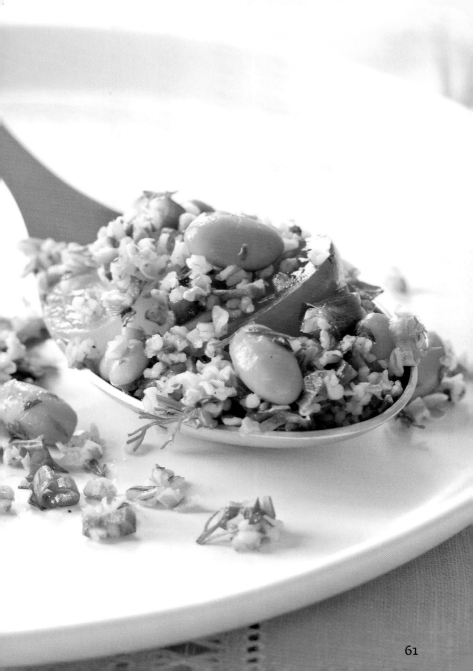

take two:

Edamame vs.

Give your meal a nutritional boost by adding either of these healthy legumes. Peas will lend a sweet flavor, while edamame contributes a crisp nuttiness. Try them as a side dish on their own, or toss into salads or pasta dishes. (Add legumes to pasta water during the last few minutes of boiling for easy cooking.) While soybeans contain almost twice the calories, due to their abundant heart-healthy fats, they also pack three times the satiating protein and more potassium. Both have about the same amount of fiber per serving.

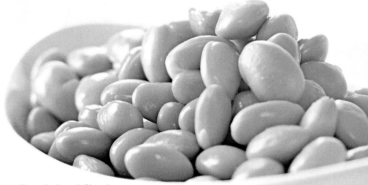

Edamame (Green Soybeans) (½ cup)
- 90 calories
- 9 grams protein
- 5 grams fat (1 gram saturated)
- 3.6 grams fiber
- 403 milligrams potassium

English Peas

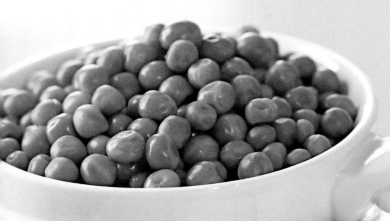

English Peas (½ cup)
- 59   calories
- 3.9 grams protein
- 0.3 grams fat (0.1 gram saturated)
- 3.7 grams fiber
- 177 milligrams potassium

Did you Know? **One serving of edamame contains 9 grams of protein to help you feel fuller longer.**

Feta and Green Onion Couscous Cakes over Tomato-Olive Salad

An authentic Greek trio of tomatoes, olives, and feta cheese accompanies these couscous cakes.

1/3 cup uncooked whole-wheat couscous
1/2 cup boiling water
1/4 cup (1 ounce) crumbled feta cheese
3 tablespoons egg substitute
2 tablespoons finely chopped green onions
1/8 teaspoon freshly ground black pepper
2 teaspoons olive oil

Cooking spray
2/3 cup chopped seeded tomato
2 tablespoons chopped pitted kalamata olives
2 tablespoons chopped fresh parsley
2 teaspoons red wine vinegar
1/2 teaspoon olive oil
1/8 teaspoon freshly ground black pepper
3 cups gourmet salad greens

1. Place couscous in a medium bowl; stir in 1/2 cup boiling water. Cover and let stand 5 minutes or until liquid is absorbed. Fluff with a fork. Cool slightly. Add cheese and next 3 ingredients. Heat 2 teaspoons oil in a large nonstick skillet coated with cooking spray over medium-high heat. Spoon about 1/3 cup couscous mixture into 4 mounds in pan. Lightly press with a spatula to flatten to 1/2 inch. Cook 2 minutes or until lightly browned. Coat tops of cakes with cooking spray. Carefully turn cakes over; cook 2 minutes or until heated.

2. Combine tomato and next 5 ingredients. Arrange 1 1/2 cups greens on each of 2 plates. Arrange 2 cakes over greens; top each serving with 1/2 cup tomato mixture. **YIELD:** 2 servings.

CALORIES 289; FAT 14g (sat 3.6g, mono 8.1g, poly 1.8g); PROTEIN 10.7g; CARB 30.6g; FIBER 4.4g; CHOL 13mg; IRON 2.7mg; SODIUM 478mg; CALC 154mg

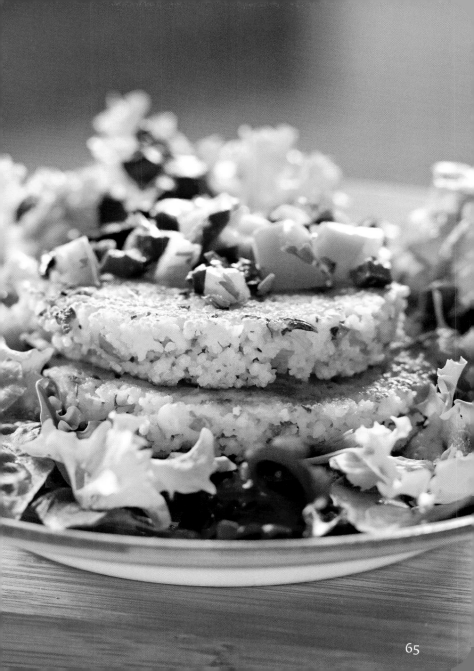

Falafel with Avocado Spread

- 1 (15-ounce) can pinto beans, rinsed and drained
- ¹/₂ cup (2 ounces) shredded Monterey Jack cheese
- ¹/₄ cup finely crushed baked tortilla chips (about ³/₄ ounce)
- 2 tablespoons finely chopped green onions
- 1 tablespoon finely chopped cilantro
- ¹/₈ teaspoon ground cumin
- 1 large egg white
- 1¹/₂ teaspoons canola oil
- ¹/₄ cup mashed peeled avocado
- 2 tablespoons finely chopped tomato
- 1 tablespoon finely chopped red onion
- 2 tablespoons fat-free sour cream
- 1 teaspoon fresh lime juice
- ¹/₈ teaspoon salt
- 2 (6-inch) pitas, each cut in half crosswise
- 4 thin red onion slices, separated into rings

Microgreens or baby greens

1. Place pinto beans in a medium bowl; partially mash with a fork. Add cheese and next 5 ingredients; stir until well combined. Shape bean mixture into 4 (¹/₂-inch-thick) oval patties.

2. Heat oil in a large nonstick skillet over medium-high heat. Add patties to pan; cook 3 minutes on each side or until patties are browned and thoroughly heated.

3. Combine avocado and next 5 ingredients, stirring well. Place 1 patty in each pita half. Spread about 2 tablespoons avocado spread over patty in each pita half; top with onions and greens.

YIELD: 4 servings (serving size: 1 stuffed pita half).

CALORIES 281; FAT 9.5g (sat 3.4g, mono 3.9g, poly 1.5g); PROTEIN 12.2g; CARB 37.4g; FIBER 5.9g; CHOL 13mg; IRON 2.4mg; SODIUM 625mg; CALC 188mg

RECIPE BENEFIT: high-fiber

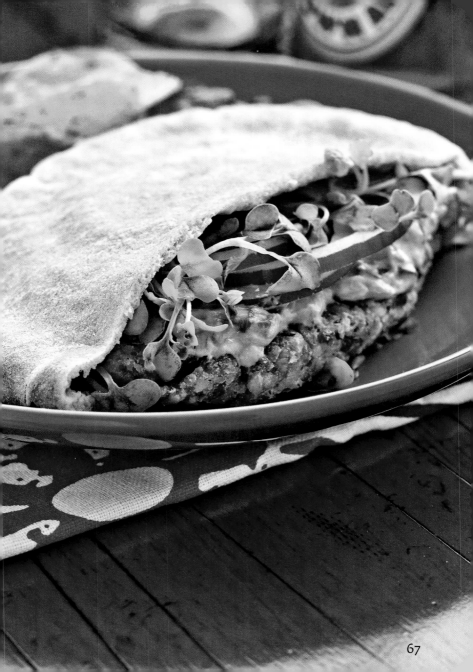

Grilled Vegetable Pitas with Goat Cheese and Pesto Mayo

8   (4-inch) portobello mushroom caps (about 1 pound)
4   medium red bell peppers, quartered
2   medium Vidalia or other sweet onions, each cut into 4 slices (about 1¼ pounds)
Cooking spray
½   teaspoon kosher salt
¼   teaspoon freshly ground black pepper
1½ tablespoons balsamic vinegar
¼   cup reduced-fat mayonnaise
1   tablespoon commercial pesto
2   (6-inch) whole-wheat pitas, each cut in half
4   leaf lettuce leaves
½   cup (2 ounces) crumbled goat cheese

1. Prepare grill.

2. Arrange mushrooms, gill sides up; bell pepper quarters; and onion slices on a baking sheet. Coat vegetables with cooking spray. Sprinkle evenly with salt and black pepper. Drizzle vinegar over mushrooms. Place vegetables on grill rack; grill 5 minutes on each side or until tender.

3. Combine mayonnaise and pesto.

4. Spread 1 tablespoon mayonnaise mixture into each pita half. Stuff each pita half with 1 lettuce leaf, vegetable mixture, and 2 tablespoons cheese. Serve immediately. YIELD: 4 servings (servings size: 1 stuffed pita half).

CALORIES 220; FAT 7.3g (sat 2.5g, mono 1.6g, poly 1.6g); PROTEIN 8.9g; CARB 33.7g; FIBER 5.8g; CHOL 7mg; IRON 2.1mg; SODIUM 505mg; CALC 62mg

RECIPE BENEFIT: high-fiber

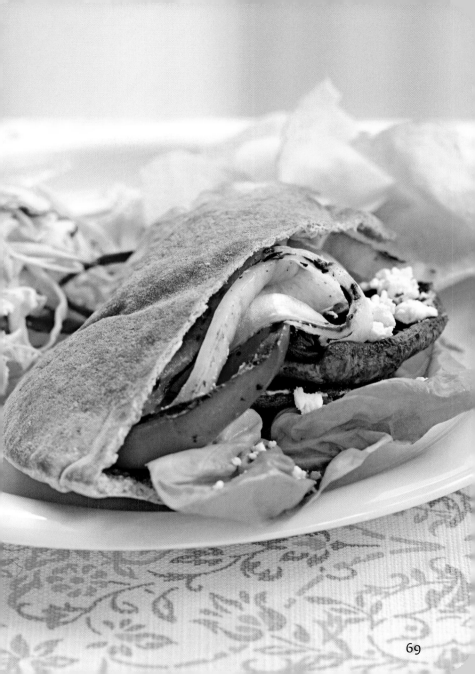

Black Bean Soup

Cumin and fiery serrano chile infuse this simple soup as it cooks, and a dollop of sour cream provides a refreshing foil for the spicy flavors. For less heat, seed the chile first or use a milder pepper, such as jalapeño. You can also omit the chile, if you prefer.

1 pound dried black beans	1 serrano chile, finely chopped
4 cups fat-free, less-sodium chicken broth	2 tablespoons fresh lime juice
2 cups chopped onion	1 teaspoon kosher salt
1 cup water	¼ cup chopped fresh cilantro
1 tablespoon ground cumin	3 tablespoons reduced-fat sour cream
3 bay leaves	Cilantro sprigs (optional)

1. Sort and wash beans; place in a large bowl. Cover with water to 2 inches above beans; cover and let stand 8 hours. Drain.

2. Combine beans, broth, and next 5 ingredients in an electric slow cooker. Cover and cook on LOW 10 hours. Discard bay leaves. Stir in juice and salt. Ladle 1½ cups soup into each of 6 bowls; sprinkle each with 2 teaspoons chopped cilantro. Top each serving with 1½ teaspoons sour cream. Garnish with cilantro sprigs, if desired. **YIELD:** 6 servings.

CALORIES 288; FAT 2.3g (sat 0.9g, mono 0.4g, poly 0.5g); PROTEIN 18.5g; CARB 50g; FIBER 17.5g; CHOL 2.9mg; IRON 4.6mg; SODIUM 581mg; CALC 87mg

RECIPE BENEFITS: low-fat; high-fiber

CHOICE INGREDIENT: *Cumin*

Cumin is an aromatic member of the parsley family with a pungent, nutty flavor. Its earliest recorded use comes from ancient Greece, and it is still used in many Mediterranean dishes. It also appears in Indian curries and garam masala, Mexican chili powders and salsa, Thai marinades, North African Berber spice mixes, and European sausages. In this dish, it takes on a Latin-American role. Cumin is typically found ground, but you can also buy the seeds whole.

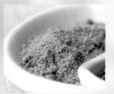

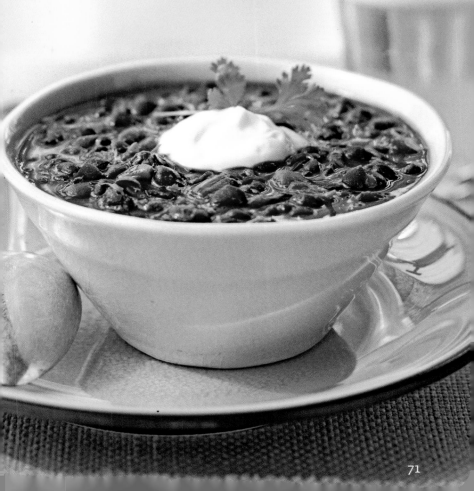

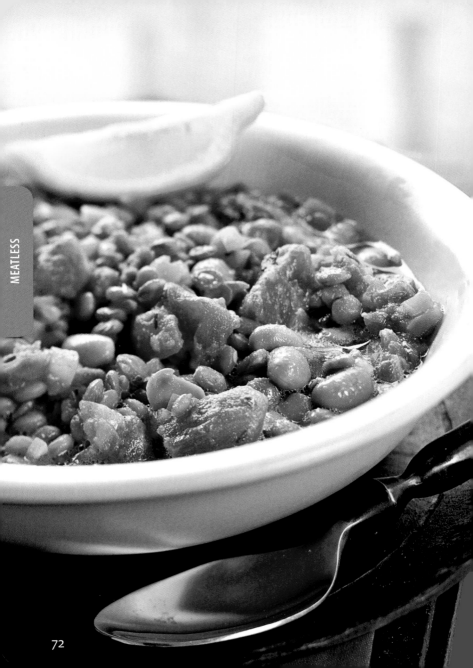

Lentil-Edamame Stew

Fava beans are traditional in this stew, which we updated with edamame. You can also substitute green peas for the edamame, if you like. Scoop up the thick stew with a warm pita. Halve the portion if you'd like to serve this as a hearty side dish.

1   cup dried lentils
¾   cup frozen shelled edamame (green soybeans)
2   tablespoons olive oil
1½   cups minced red onion
3   garlic cloves, minced
1   (14.5-ounce) can diced tomatoes, undrained
6   tablespoons fresh lemon juice

1   tablespoon chopped fresh parsley
1   tablespoon chopped fresh mint
½   teaspoon salt
½   teaspoon ground cumin
⅛   teaspoon ground red pepper
⅛   teaspoon ground cinnamon
Dash of ground cloves
Lemon wedges (optional)

1. Place lentils in a large saucepan; cover with water to 2 inches above lentils. Bring to a boil; cover, reduce heat, and simmer 20 minutes or until tender. Drain well, and set aside.

2. Place edamame in a small saucepan; cover with water to 2 inches above edamame. Bring to a boil; cook 2 minutes or until edamame are tender. Remove from heat; drain well.

3. Heat oil in a Dutch oven over medium-high heat. Add onion, garlic, and tomatoes to pan; sauté 6 minutes or until onion is translucent, stirring often. Stir in lentils, edamame, lemon juice, and remaining ingredients. Cook 2 minutes or until thoroughly heated, stirring often. Garnish with lemon wedges, if desired.

YIELD: 4 servings (serving size: about 1 cup).

CALORIES 320; FAT 8g (sat 1.1g, mono 5.2g, poly 1.4g); PROTEIN 18.6g; CARB 48.4g; FIBER 10.7g; CHOL 0mg; IRON 5.7mg; SODIUM 432mg; CALC 59mg

RECIPE BENEFITS: healthy fats; low-fat; high-fiber; low-sodium

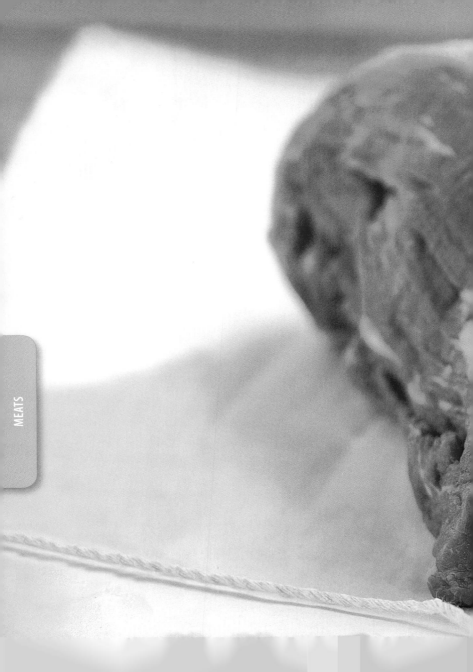

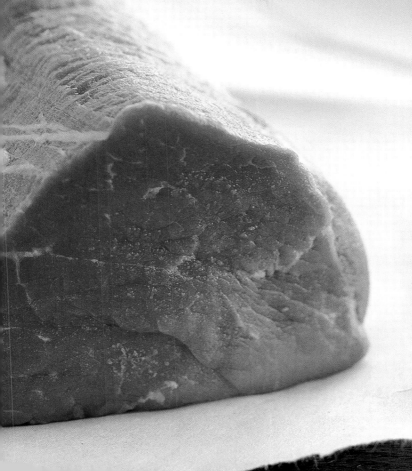

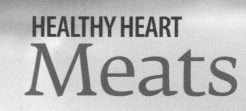

HEALTHY HEART
Meats

Our Favorite Cuts of Beef

Two cuts show up repeatedly in our recipes: tenderloin and flank steak. Tenderloin is the most tender, luxurious cut you can buy, and it's very lean. Roasted whole, it's the ideal entrée for a celebratory dinner. Cut into filets and pan-seared, it's a superb supper for two. Cut into cubes, it makes outstanding kebabs on the grill.

Flank steak is one of those tough-but-flavorful cuts, and it has a little more fat than tenderloin. Its flat shape and coarse grain absorb flavors quickly, making it a good candidate for marinades.

Here are four lesser-known budget-friendly lean cuts:

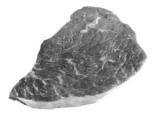

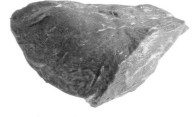

Bottom round steak, aka Western griller. Boneless and quick cooking; best marinated to help tenderize.

Shoulder tender, aka butcher's steak, petite filet, chuck shoulder steak. Resembles pork loin; slice into medallions and grill.

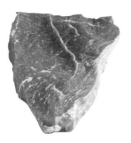

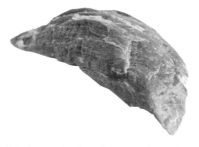

Shoulder center steak, aka ranch steak, shoulder grill steak. Moderately tender; serve whole or sliced.

Tri-tip steak, aka sirloin triangle tip. Comes from the bottom sirloin; rich flavor; affordable. Roast or grill whole, and then slice.

Grilled Flank Steak Soft Tacos with Avocado-Lime Salsa

1 tablespoon chili powder
2 teaspoons grated lime rind
$^{1}/_{2}$ teaspoon salt
$^{1}/_{2}$ teaspoon chipotle chile powder
$^{1}/_{4}$ teaspoon freshly ground black pepper
1 (1-pound) flank steak, trimmed
Cooking spray
1 cup diced peeled avocado
$^{3}/_{4}$ cup finely chopped tomato
$^{1}/_{3}$ cup finely chopped Vidalia or other sweet onion

$^{1}/_{4}$ cup chopped fresh cilantro
$^{1}/_{2}$ teaspoon grated lime rind
2 tablespoons fresh lime juice
$^{1}/_{4}$ teaspoon salt
$^{1}/_{4}$ teaspoon hot pepper sauce (such as Tabasco)
8 (6-inch) corn tortillas
2 cups very thinly sliced green cabbage

1. To prepare steak, combine first 5 ingredients in a small bowl. Score a diamond pattern on both sides of steak. Rub chili powder mixture evenly over steak. Cover and chill 1 hour.

2. Prepare grill to medium-high heat.

3. Place steak on grill rack coated with cooking spray; grill 8 minutes on each side or until desired degree of doneness. Remove from heat; let stand 10 minutes. Cut steak diagonally across grain into thin slices.

4. To prepare salsa, combine avocado and next 7 ingredients in a medium bowl.

5. Warm tortillas according to package directions. Spoon steak mixture evenly over each of 8 tortillas. Top each taco with $^{1}/_{4}$ cup salsa and $^{1}/_{4}$ cup cabbage. **YIELD:** 4 servings (serving size: 2 tacos).

CALORIES 353; FAT 16g (sat 4.3g, mono 7.6g, poly 1.7g); PROTEIN 27.9g; CARB 27.7g; FIBER 6.8g; CHOL 40mg; IRON 2.5mg; SODIUM 593mg; CALC 78mg

RECIPE BENEFIT: high-fiber

Mongolian Beef

This spicy Asian favorite gets its flavor from hoisin sauce and dark sesame oil. Hoisin sauce is a versatile, sweet-and-spicy condiment that is used in Chinese cooking and dining much the same way Westerners use ketchup. The dark sesame oil imparts a distinctive nutty taste and aroma to the dish. Serve with boil-in-bag jasmine rice and steamed snow peas.

1 (1-pound) flank steak, trimmed and cut into thin slices	1 teaspoon bottled minced roasted garlic
Butter-flavored cooking spray	2 teaspoons dark sesame oil
⅓ cup hoisin sauce	½ teaspoon crushed red pepper
2 tablespoons water	4 green onions
2 teaspoons minced peeled fresh ginger	

1. Heat a large nonstick skillet over medium-high heat. Coat steak with cooking spray. Add steak to pan; cook 3 minutes or until browned and liquid has almost evaporated, stirring occasionally.

2. While steak cooks, combine hoisin sauce and next 5 ingredients in a small bowl. Cut onions crosswise into 1-inch pieces. Add sauce mixture and onions to meat in pan; cook 1 to 2 minutes or until sauce is slightly reduced (do not overcook meat). Serve immediately. **YIELD:** 4 servings (serving size: about ½ cup).

CALORIES 240; FAT 10g (sat 2.8g, mono 3.4g, poly 2.6g); PROTEIN 25.5g; CARB 11.1g; FIBER 1.1g; CHOL 38mg; IRON 2.2mg; SODIUM 410mg; CALC 45mg

KITCHEN TIP: Snow peas are at their best when steamed. To steam them, cook, covered, in a steamer basket or on a rack above boiling water 2 to 3 minutes.

MEATS

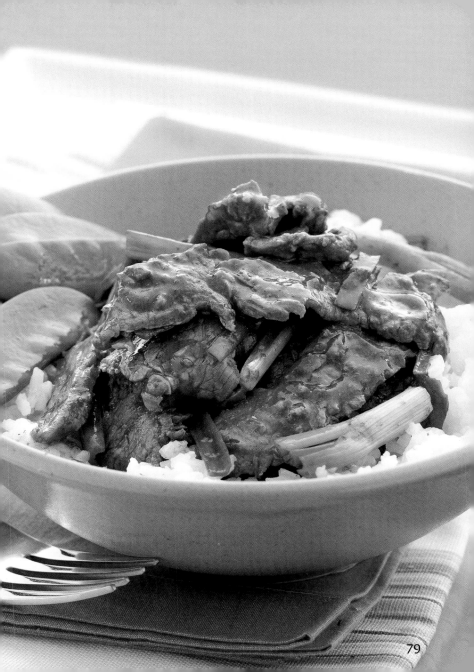

Roasted Flank Steak with Olive Oil–Herb Rub

To serve two, use two (four-ounce) beef tenderloin steaks instead of flank steak, reduce the herbs to $1/2$ teaspoon each, and omit the broth. Finish the tenderloin in the oven for two minutes instead of 10.

- 1 teaspoon chopped fresh thyme
- 1 teaspoon chopped fresh oregano
- 1 teaspoon chopped fresh parsley
- 2 teaspoons olive oil
- $1/8$ teaspoon grated lemon rind
- 1 garlic clove, minced
- $1/2$ teaspoon salt
- $1/4$ teaspoon freshly ground black pepper
- 1 ($1^1/2$-pound) flank steak, trimmed
- Cooking spray
- $1/4$ cup dry red wine
- $1/4$ cup fat-free, less-sodium beef broth
- Thyme springs (optional)

1. Preheat oven to 400°.

2. Combine first 6 ingredients in a small bowl; set aside.

3. Sprinkle salt and pepper over steak. Heat a large ovenproof skillet over medium-high heat. Coat pan with cooking spray. Add steak to pan; cook 1 minute on each side or until browned. Add wine and broth; cook 1 minute. Spread herb mixture over steak; place pan in oven. Bake at 400° for 10 minutes or until desired degree of doneness. Let stand 10 minutes before cutting steak diagonally across the grain into thin slices. Serve with pan sauce. Garnish with fresh thyme sprigs, if desired. YIELD: 6 servings (serving size: 3 ounces steak and about 1 tablespoon sauce).

CALORIES 167; FAT 7g (sat 2.5g, mono 3.3g, poly 0.4g); PROTEIN 23.9g; CARB 0.5g; FIBER 0.1g; CHOL 37mg; IRON 1.6mg; SODIUM 266mg; CALC 21mg

KITCHEN TIP: Freeze tablespoons of leftover ingredients such as tomato paste, broths, chipotle chiles, and pesto in ice cube trays. Once solid, pop them out and store them in zip-top plastic bags.

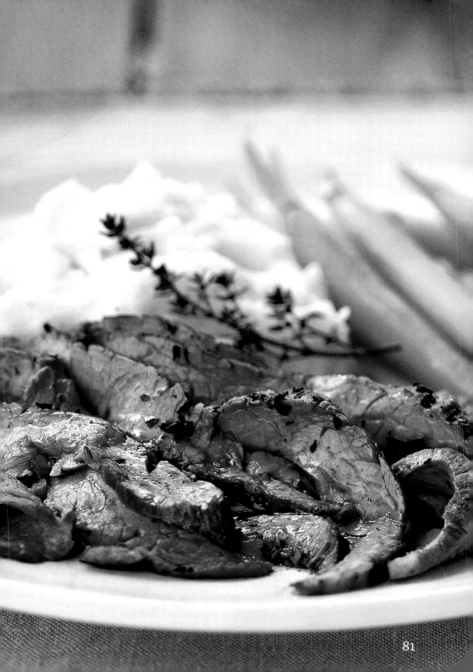

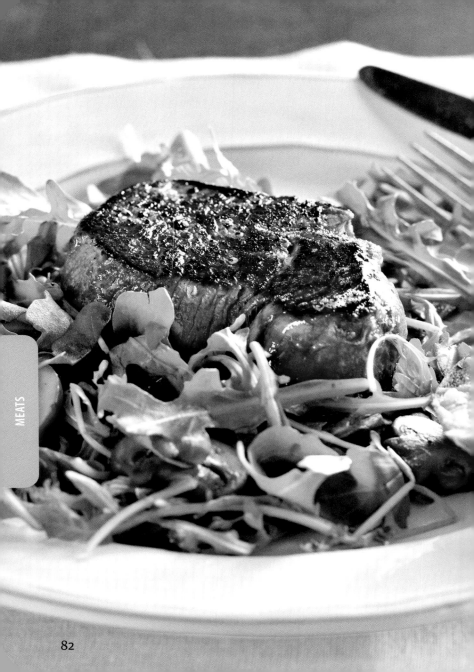

Filet Mignon with Arugula Salad

Arugula, a peppery salad green, makes a tasty bed for pan-seared steak. Asiago garlic bread is a fitting accompaniment. To make, combine 1 tablespoon olive oil and 1 minced garlic clove; brush evenly over 4 (1-inch-thick) French bread slices. Top each bread slice with 1 tablespoon grated Asiago cheese. Broil 2 minutes or until cheese melts and bread is toasted.

Cooking spray
4 (4-ounce) beef tenderloin steaks, trimmed
½ teaspoon salt, divided
¼ teaspoon black pepper, divided
2 teaspoons butter

½ cup prechopped red onion
1 (8-ounce) package presliced cremini mushrooms
2 tablespoons fresh lemon juice
1 (5-ounce) bag baby arugula

1. Heat a large nonstick skillet over medium-high heat. Coat pan with cooking spray. Sprinkle beef with ¼ teaspoon salt and ⅛ teaspoon pepper. Add beef to pan; cook 4 minutes on each side or until desired degree of doneness. Remove beef from pan; keep warm.

2. Melt butter in pan; coat pan with cooking spray. Add remaining ¼ teaspoon salt, remaining ⅛ teaspoon pepper, red onion, and mushrooms to pan; sauté 4 minutes or until mushrooms release their liquid. Combine juice and arugula in a large bowl. Add mushroom mixture to arugula mixture; toss gently to combine. Arrange 1½ cups salad mixture on each of 4 plates; top each serving with 1 steak. **YIELD:** 4 servings.

CALORIES 191; FAT 8.9g (sat 3.8g, mono 3.1g, poly 0.5g); PROTEIN 20.5g; CARB 7g; FIBER 1.8g; CHOL 59mg; IRON 3.3mg; SODIUM 349mg; CALC 72mg

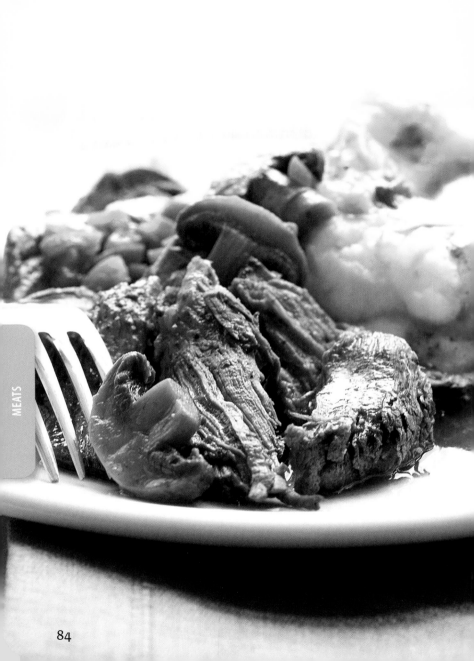

Slow-Cooker Beef Pot Roast

Pair this homestyle favorite with mashed potatoes to soak up the sauce. Leftover meat makes great hot roast beef sandwiches the next day.

1 (8-ounce) package presliced mushrooms
1 (8-ounce) container refrigerated prechopped green bell pepper
Cooking spray
¼ cup plus 2 tablespoons ketchup
¼ cup water
1 tablespoon Worcestershire sauce
½ teaspoon black pepper
¼ teaspoon salt
2 pounds boneless shoulder pot roast

1. Place mushrooms and bell pepper in a 3½- to 4-quart electric slow cooker coated with cooking spray.

2. Combine ketchup and next 4 ingredients in a small bowl, stirring until blended.

3. Heat a large nonstick skillet over medium-high heat. Coat pan and roast with cooking spray. Cook 3 minutes on each side or until browned. Place roast over vegetables in cooker; pour ketchup mixture over roast. Cover and cook on HIGH for 1 hour. Reduce heat to LOW; cook 6 to 7 hours or until roast is very tender. Serve vegetables and sauce over roast. YIELD: 6 servings (serving size: 3 ounces beef and ½ cup vegetables and sauce).

CALORIES 228; FAT 8g (sat 2g, mono 3.1g, poly 0.1g); PROTEIN 31.3g; CARB 7.4g; FIBER 1.1g; CHOL 89mg; IRON 4.2mg; SODIUM 397mg; CALC 21mg

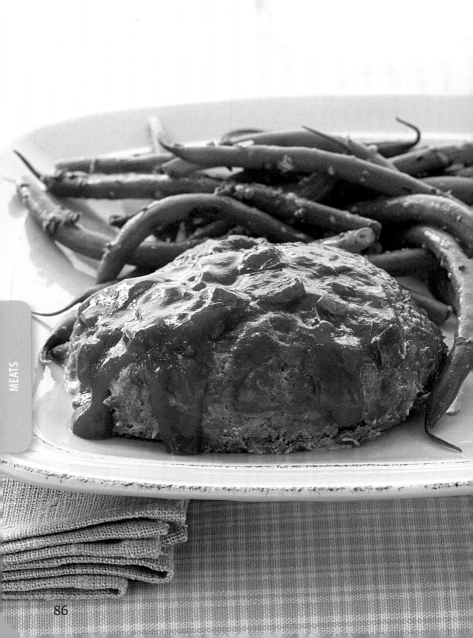

Individual Salsa Meat Loaves

Making meat loaf in single-serving portions reduces the cooking time by half and keeps the meat juicy.

2 **large egg whites**
$^1/_3$ **cup quick-cooking oats**
$^1/_2$ **cup plus 2 tablespoons chipotle salsa, divided**
$^1/_4$ **cup ketchup, divided**
1 **pound ground beef, extra lean**
Cooking spray

1. Preheat oven to 350°.
2. Combine egg whites in a large bowl, stirring well with a whisk. Stir in oats, $^1/_2$ cup salsa, and 2 tablespoons ketchup. Add beef; mix well. Divide beef mixture into 4 equal portions, shaping each into an oval-shaped loaf. Coat a foil-lined rimmed baking sheet with cooking spray. Place loaves on prepared pan.
3. Bake at 350° for 30 minutes or until done.
4. Combine remaining 2 tablespoons salsa and remaining 2 tablespoons ketchup in a small bowl; spread mixture evenly over loaves. **YIELD:** 4 servings (serving size: 1 meat loaf).

CALORIES 190; FAT 6g (sat 2.1g, mono 2.1g, poly 0.7g); PROTEIN 25g; CARB 10.9g; FIBER 1.7g; CHOL 60mg; IRON 2.2mg; SODIUM 548mg; CALC 7mg

INGREDIENT TIP: To accurately gauge the amount of fat in ground beef, look at the percentages. If the package is labeled "80% lean," that means it's 20% fat. In addition to ground chuck (20% fat), round (15% fat), and sirloin (10% fat), you may also find lean ground beef (7%) and extra-lean ground beef (5%).

Pork Chops with Mustard Cream Sauce

Using fat-free half-and-half gives this dish a creamy, rich flavor that fat-free milk can't. Sprinkle the finished dish with chopped fresh parsley, if desired.

4 (4-ounce) boneless center-cut loin pork chops (¹/₂ inch thick)	²/₃ cup fat-free half-and-half
¹/₂ teaspoon salt	1 tablespoon Dijon mustard
¹/₄ teaspoon black pepper	2 teaspoons lemon juice
Cooking spray	Chopped fresh parsley (optional)
¹/₂ cup fat-free, less-sodium chicken broth	

1. Sprinkle both sides of pork with salt and pepper.

2. Heat a large nonstick skillet over medium-high heat. Coat pan with cooking spray. Add pork, and cook 4 to 5 minutes on each side or until lightly browned and done. Transfer pork to a serving plate, and keep warm.

3. Add broth to pan, scraping pan to loosen browned bits. Stir in half-and-half, mustard, and lemon juice. Reduce heat, and simmer, uncovered, 6 minutes or until sauce is slightly thick. Spoon sauce over pork; sprinkle with parsley, if desired. YIELD: 4 servings (serving size: 1 pork chop and 2 tablespoons sauce).

CALORIES 193; FAT 6.4g (sat 2.3g; mono 2.7g; poly 1.2g); PROTEIN 24.3g; CARB 5.2g; FIBER 0g; CHOL 65mg; IRON 0.7mg; SODIUM 539mg; CALC 52mg

MEATS

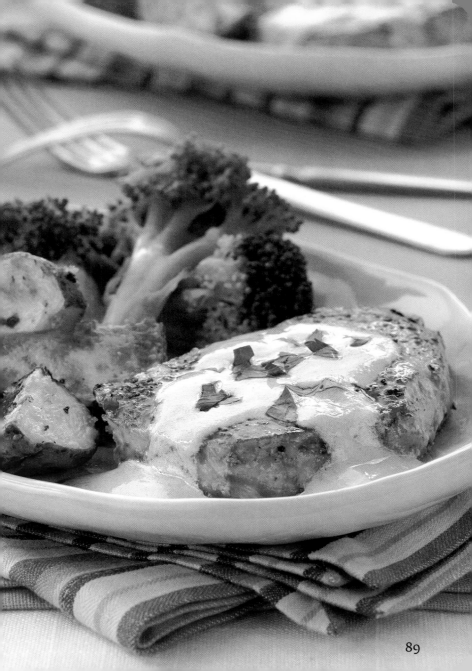

Prepare Pork Tenderloin

When preparing pork tenderloin, remove the silver skin, which is the thin, shiny membrane that runs along the surface of the meat. Leaving it on can cause the tenderloin to toughen and lose shape during cooking.

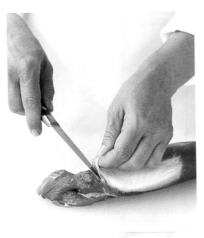 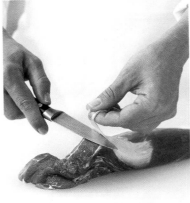

MEATS

1. Stretch the membrane with one hand so it's tight, and use your other hand to slip the tip of the knife underneath the silver skin.

2. Slowly slice back and forth, angling the sharp edge of the blade up, rather than down, through the meat. Continue until all the silver skin is removed; discard the skin.

Grilled Pork with Blackberry-Sage Sauce

If your blackberries are particularly sweet or tart, adjust the amount of sugar in the sauce accordingly by $1/2$ teaspoon or so to find the right balance.

Cooking spray
2 tablespoons minced shallots
3 cups fresh blackberries (about 1 pound)
$1/2$ teaspoon chopped fresh sage
1 (14-ounce) can fat-free, less-sodium chicken broth
2 tablespoons balsamic vinegar
$1^1/2$ teaspoons sugar
1 tablespoon butter
$3/4$ teaspoon kosher salt, divided
1 teaspoon black pepper
1 ($1^1/2$-pound) pork tenderloin, trimmed

1. Prepare grill to medium heat.

2. Heat a medium saucepan over medium heat. Coat pan with cooking spray. Add shallots to pan; cook 3 minutes or until tender, stirring occasionally. Add blackberries, sage, and broth; bring to a boil. Reduce heat, and simmer 20 minutes or until blackberries break down. Press blackberry mixture through a fine sieve over a bowl; discard solids. Return liquid to pan. Stir in vinegar and sugar; bring to a boil. Cook until reduced to $3/4$ cup (about 9 minutes); remove from heat. Stir in butter and $1/4$ teaspoon salt, stirring until butter melts. Keep warm.

3. Sprinkle remaining $1/2$ teaspoon salt and pepper over pork. Place pork on grill rack coated with cooking spray; cover and grill 20 minutes or until a thermometer registers 155° (slightly pink), turning pork occasionally. Let stand 10 minutes. Cut crosswise into $1/4$-inch-thick slices. Serve with blackberry sauce. YIELD: 6 servings (serving size: about 3 ounces pork and 2 tablespoons sauce).

CALORIES 199; FAT 6.1g (sat 2.6g, mono 2.3g, poly 0.7g); PROTEIN 25.3g; CARB 10g; FIBER 4g; CHOL 79mg; IRON 2mg; SODIUM 439mg; CALC 32mg

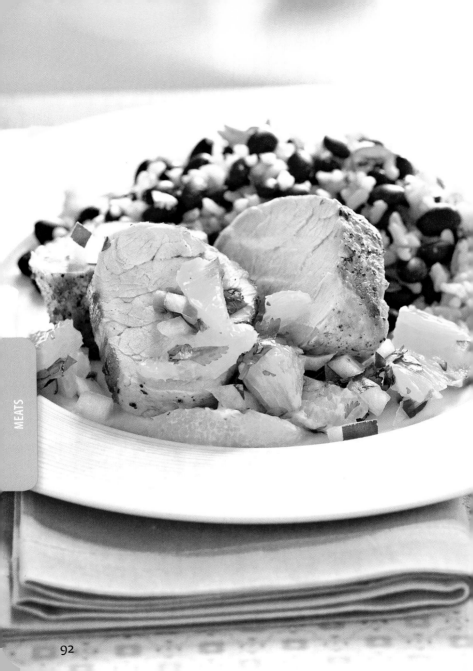

Roasted Pork Tenderloin with Orange and Red Onion Salsa

A quick and hearty rice-and-beans side dish complements the roast. To make, cook 1 (10-ounce) package frozen long-grain brown rice (such as Birds Eye Steamfresh) according to package directions. Combine cooked rice, 1 cup rinsed and drained canned black beans, 1 tablespoon chopped fresh cilantro, $\frac{1}{4}$ teaspoon salt, $\frac{1}{4}$ teaspoon ground cumin, and $\frac{1}{8}$ teaspoon chili powder.

- 1 tablespoon canola oil
- 1 (1-pound) pork tenderloin, trimmed
- $\frac{1}{2}$ teaspoon salt, divided
- $\frac{1}{2}$ teaspoon freshly ground black pepper, divided
- 1 cup coarsely chopped orange sections (about 2 oranges)
- $\frac{1}{2}$ cup diced red onion
- $\frac{1}{4}$ cup chopped fresh cilantro
- 2 tablespoons fresh lime juice
- 2 teaspoons minced seeded jalapeño pepper
- 1 teaspoon minced garlic

1. Preheat oven to 450°.

2. Heat oil in a large ovenproof skillet over medium-high heat. Sprinkle pork evenly with $\frac{1}{4}$ teaspoon salt and $\frac{1}{4}$ teaspoon black pepper. Add pork to pan; cook 2 minutes on each side or until lightly browned. Transfer pan to oven. Bake at 450° for 17 minutes or until a thermometer registers 160°. Let stand 5 minutes; cut across grain into $\frac{1}{2}$-inch-thick slices.

3. Combine remaining $\frac{1}{4}$ teaspoon salt, remaining $\frac{1}{4}$ teaspoon black pepper, oranges, and remaining ingredients. Serve salsa with pork. **YIELD:** 4 servings (serving size: 3 ounces pork and about $\frac{1}{4}$ cup salsa).

CALORIES 220; FAT 8.5g (sat 2g, mono 4.1g, poly 1.5g); PROTEIN 23.6g; CARB 13.6g; FIBER 4g; CHOL 65mg; IRON 1.5mg; SODIUM 342mg; CALC 44mg

Warm Spinach Salad with Pork and Pears

A loaf of whole-grain or sesame seed bread completes the dinner.
Blue cheese balances the sweetness of the pears and raisins;
choose a premium variety such as Maytag for more intensity.

Cooking spray

1 (1-pound) pork tenderloin, trimmed and cut crosswise into 12 slices

$1/2$ teaspoon salt, divided

$1/4$ teaspoon black pepper, divided

3 tablespoons water

3 tablespoons sherry vinegar or red wine vinegar

1 tablespoon extra-virgin olive oil

2 cups thinly sliced Anjou or Bartlett pear (about 2)

$1/4$ cup golden raisins

1 (5-ounce) package baby spinach

2 tablespoons crumbled blue cheese

1. Heat a large nonstick skillet over medium-high heat. Coat pan with cooking spray. Sprinkle pork evenly with $1/4$ teaspoon salt and $1/8$ teaspoon pepper. Add pork to pan; cook 4 minutes on each side or until browned.

2. Combine remaining $1/4$ teaspoon salt, remaining $1/8$ teaspoon pepper, 3 tablespoons water, vinegar, and oil in a small bowl, stirring with a whisk.

3. Combine pear, raisins, and spinach in a large bowl; toss well. Arrange 2 cups spinach mixture on each of 4 plates, and drizzle evenly with vinegar mixture. Top each serving with 3 pork slices and $1^1/2$ teaspoons cheese. **YIELD:** 4 servings.

CALORIES 296; FAT 10.1g (sat 3g, mono 4.8g, poly 0.8g); PROTEIN 25.5g; CARB 27.4g; FIBER 4.5g; CHOL 68mg; IRON 2.8mg; SODIUM 471mg; CALC 117mg

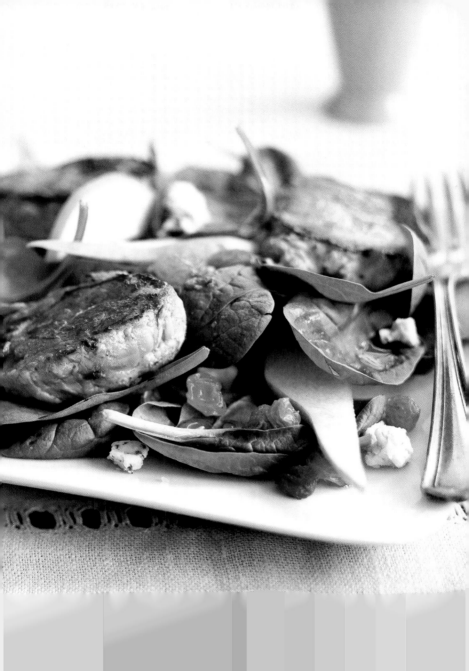

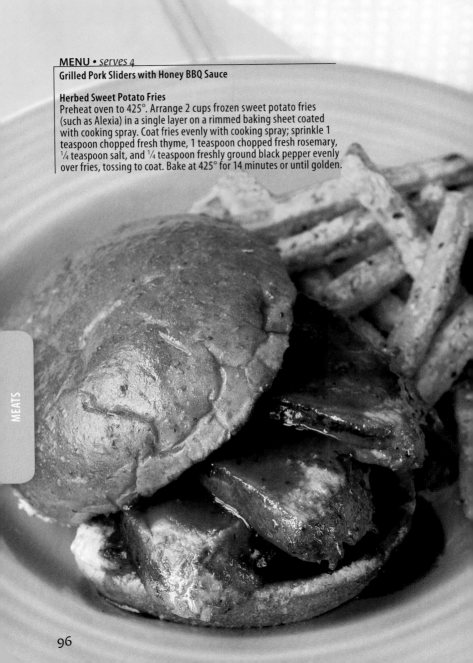

MENU • *serves 4*

Grilled Pork Sliders with Honey BBQ Sauce

Herbed Sweet Potato Fries
Preheat oven to 425°. Arrange 2 cups frozen sweet potato fries (such as Alexia) in a single layer on a rimmed baking sheet coated with cooking spray. Coat fries evenly with cooking spray; sprinkle 1 teaspoon chopped fresh thyme, 1 teaspoon chopped fresh rosemary, ¼ teaspoon salt, and ¼ teaspoon freshly ground black pepper evenly over fries, tossing to coat. Bake at 425° for 14 minutes or until golden.

MEATS

Grilled Pork Sliders with Honey BBQ Sauce

Crisp on the outside, soft on the inside, Herbed Sweet Potato Fries (recipe at left) are the perfect side to pair with a barbecue pork sandwich. We guarantee you can't eat just one. And that's a good thing: Sweet potatoes are rich in beta carotene, vitamin C, and vitamin E.

$^1\!/_2$ **cup bottled barbecue sauce (such as Sticky Fingers Memphis Original)**

2 **tablespoons dark rum (such as Myers's)**

2 **tablespoons honey**

1 **(1-pound) pork tenderloin, trimmed**

Cooking spray

4 **(1.8-ounce) white wheat hamburger buns**

1. Prepare grill.

2. Combine barbecue sauce, rum, and honey in a medium saucepan; bring to a boil. Cook 2 minutes or until reduced to $^1\!/_2$ cup. Reserve $^1\!/_4$ cup sauce for serving. Use remaining $^1\!/_4$ cup sauce for basting.

3. Place pork on grill rack coated with cooking spray. Grill pork 8 minutes. Turn and baste pork with sauce; cook 8 minutes. Turn and baste with sauce. Cook 4 minutes or until a thermometer registers 160° (slightly pink). Let stand 5 minutes; cut into thin slices.

4. Place buns, cut sides down, on grill rack; toast 1 minute. Place 3 ounces pork on bottom half of each bun. Spoon 1 tablespoon sauce over each serving; top with remaining halves of buns.

YIELD: 4 servings (serving size: 1 sandwich).

CALORIES 319; FAT 6g (sat 1.8g, mono 1.5g, poly 1.4g); PROTEIN 27.6g; CARB 39.2g; FIBER 5.1g; CHOL 63mg; IRON 4mg; SODIUM 520mg; CALC 261mg

RECIPE BENEFITS: low-fat; high-fiber

Beef and Beer Chili

Jack and Red Pepper Quesadillas
Preheat oven to 400°. Coat 1 side of each of 4 (6-inch) whole-wheat tortillas with cooking spray. Place tortillas, coated sides down, on a large baking sheet. Sprinkle each tortilla with 2 tablespoons shredded Monterey Jack cheese, 2 tablespoons chopped bottled roasted red bell peppers, 1 tablespoon chopped cilantro, and 2 teaspoons sliced green onions. Fold each tortilla in half. Bake at 400° for 5 minutes or until cheese melts. Cut into wedges.

Mixed green salad with bottled cilantro dressing

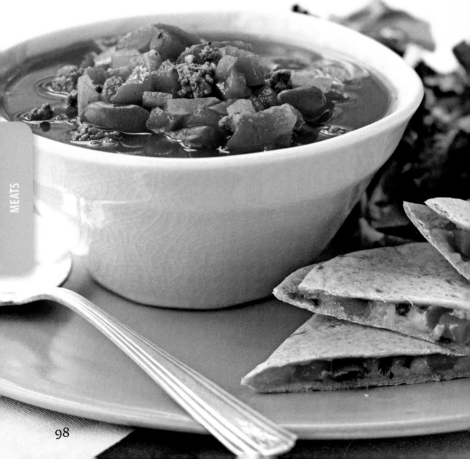

MEATS

Beef and Beer Chili

Cornmeal helps thicken the chili to a satisfying consistency.
Serve with a chilled lager.

1½ cups chopped red onion (about 1 medium)
1 cup chopped red bell pepper (about 1 small)
8 ounces extra-lean ground beef
2 garlic cloves, minced
1½ tablespoons chili powder
2 teaspoons ground cumin
1 teaspoon sugar
½ teaspoon salt
½ teaspoon dried oregano

1 (19-ounce) can red kidney beans, drained
1 (14.5-ounce) can no-salt-added diced tomatoes, undrained
1 (14-ounce) can low-sodium beef broth
1 (12-ounce) bottle beer (such as Budweiser)
1 tablespoon yellow cornmeal
1 tablespoon fresh lime juice

1. Combine first 4 ingredients in a large Dutch oven over medium-high heat. Cook 5 minutes or until beef is browned, stirring to crumble. Stir in chili powder, cumin, sugar, and salt; cook 1 minute. Add oregano and next 4 ingredients to pan; bring to a boil. Reduce heat, and simmer 15 minutes. Stir in cornmeal; cook 5 minutes. Stir in juice. **YIELD:** 4 servings (serving size: 1½ cups).

CALORIES 261; FAT 5.7g (sat 2.1g, mono 2g, poly 0.2g); PROTEIN 18.3g; CARB 30.3g; FIBER 8.3g; CHOL 30mg; IRON 3.7mg; SODIUM 799mg; CALC 74mg

RECIPE BENEFITS: low-fat; high-fiber

MAKE-AHEAD TIP: Prepare an extra batch of the chili; freeze in single-serving zip-top plastic bags for up to three months. Thaw overnight in the refrigerator, and reheat in the microwave.

Posole

The meat develops a rich, full-bodied flavor when it's cooked to a dark brown, so be sure not to stir the pork until it releases easily from the pan. Serve this fiery soup with warm flour tortillas.

Cooking spray
1 (1-pound) pork tenderloin, trimmed and cut into bite-sized pieces
2 teaspoons salt-free Southwest chipotle seasoning blend (such as Mrs. Dash)
1 (15.5-ounce) can white hominy, undrained

1 (14.5-ounce) can Mexican-style stewed tomatoes with jalapeño peppers and spices (such as Del Monte), undrained
1 cup water
¼ cup chopped fresh cilantro

1. Heat a large saucepan over medium-high heat. Coat pan with cooking spray. Sprinkle pork evenly with chipotle seasoning blend; coat evenly with cooking spray. Add pork to pan; cook 4 minutes or until browned. Stir in hominy, tomatoes, and 1 cup water. Bring to a boil; cover, reduce heat, and simmer 20 minutes or until pork is tender. Stir in cilantro. YIELD: 4 servings (serving size: 1⅓ cups).

CALORIES 233; FAT 5g (sat 1.4g, mono 1.9g, poly 0.8g); PROTEIN 24.4g; CARB 23g; FIBER 4.4g; CHOL 68mg; IRON 2.3mg; SODIUM 610mg; CALC 33mg

RECIPE BENEFIT: low-fat

CHOICE INGREDIENT: Cilantro has a pungent flavor with a faint undertone of anise. The leaves are often mistaken for flat-leaf parsley. One of the most versatile herbs, cilantro adds a distinctive taste to a variety of dishes ranging from salsas to curries to soups.

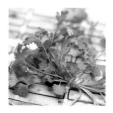

MEATS

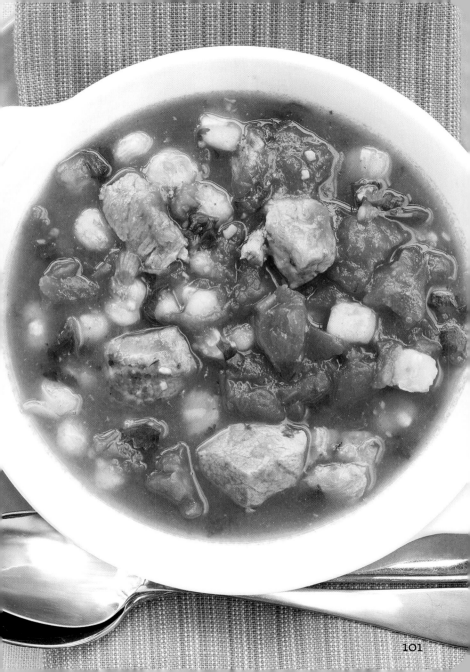

HEALTHY HEART
Poultry

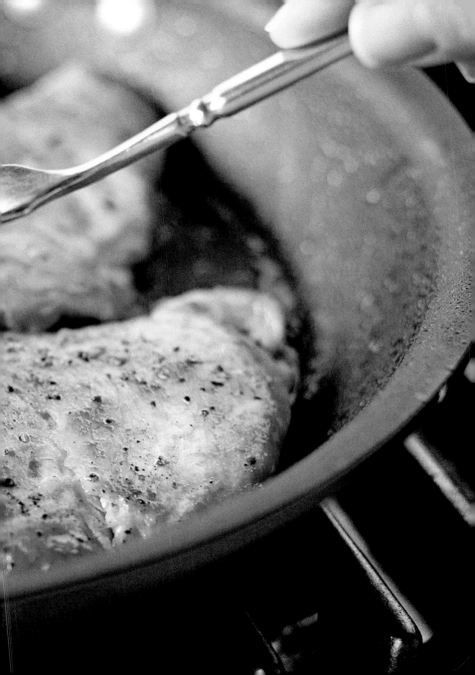

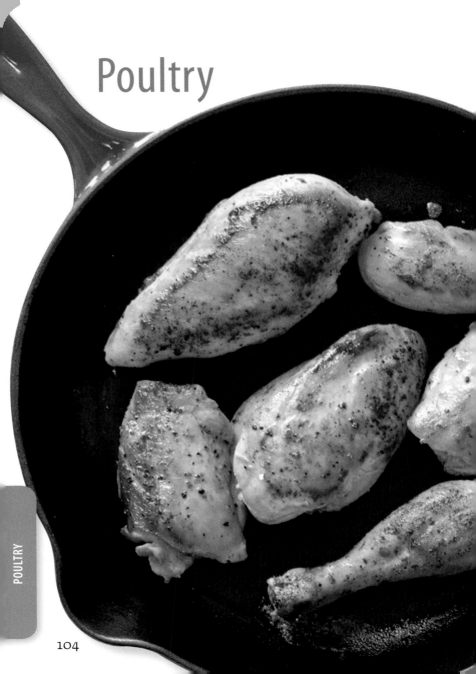

Poultry

BOTH CHICKEN AND TURKEY are traditional favorites. They're lean, flavorful, readily available, and relatively inexpensive.

LEAN CUTS

Poultry offers two types of meat: the light meat and the dark meat. The healthier of the two is the light meat, which includes the breast, because it contains less saturated fat (about 50% less) than the dark thigh, leg, and wing meat. The dark meat is dark simply because those muscles are exercised more. In nonflying birds such as turkey and chicken, the legs become dark while the breast meat stays light.

GROUND POULTRY

Poultry is an excellent alternative to beef, but not all ground varieties are the lean choices they might seem at first glance. Regular ground poultry is a mix of white meat, dark meat, and skin, which means it contains anywhere from 10% to 15% fat. It's still leaner than ground round, but it's not the healthiest choice available. Instead, look for packages labeled "ground turkey breast" or "ground chicken breast"—breast is the keyword that tells you it's lean.

LIGHT MEAT:
Four ounces has 1.4g of saturated fat.

DARK MEAT:
Four ounces has 3g of saturated fat.

ROTISSERIE CHICKEN

Rotisserie chickens are a convenient and healthy choice when the skin is removed. They're available in a variety of flavors, and all are great options because most of the added sodium will be discarded with the skin. And, as always, the light meat is better for you than the dark meat.

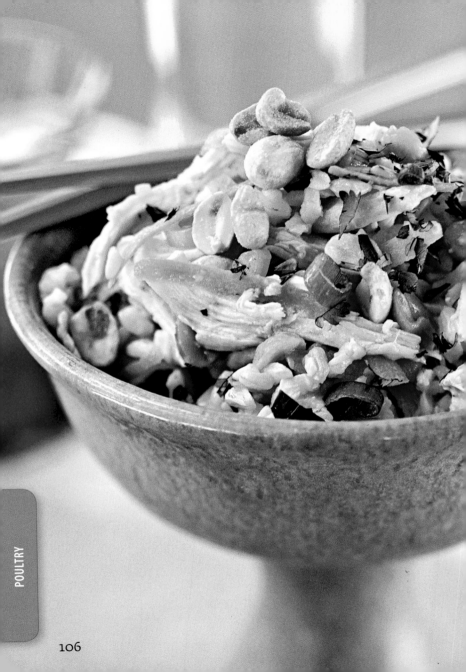

Sesame Brown Rice Salad with Shredded Chicken and Peanuts

For a burst of extra citrus flavor, serve with lime wedges.

1 cup long-grain brown rice
2 cups shredded cooked chicken breast
$^1/_2$ cup shredded carrot
$^1/_3$ cup sliced green onions
$^1/_4$ cup dry-roasted peanuts, divided

1 tablespoon chopped fresh cilantro, divided
$^1/_2$ teaspoon salt
2 tablespoons fresh lime juice
4 teaspoons canola oil
1 teaspoon dark sesame oil
2 garlic cloves, minced

1. Cook rice according to package directions, omitting salt and fat. Transfer rice to a large bowl; fluff with a fork. Cool. Add chicken, carrot, onions, 2 tablespoons peanuts, 2 teaspoons cilantro, and salt to rice; toss to combine.

2. Combine juice and remaining ingredients in a small bowl. Drizzle oil mixture over rice mixture; toss to combine. Place $1^1/_2$ cups salad on each of 4 plates. Sprinkle each serving with $1^1/_2$ teaspoons remaining peanuts and $^1/_4$ teaspoon remaining cilantro. **YIELD:** 4 servings.

CALORIES 393; FAT 13.3g (sat 2g, mono 6.3g, poly 4g); PROTEIN 27.8g; CARB 40.2g; FIBER 4g; CHOL 60mg; IRON 1.7mg; SODIUM 424mg; CALC 44mg

RECIPE BENEFIT: low-sodium

MAKE-AHEAD TIP: Grain salads are a great make-ahead option, but as they sit, the grains will absorb dressings. Adjust the seasoning just before serving by adding a bit of acid, such as fresh citrus juice or vinegar, a pinch of salt, and a grinding of black pepper. Salads are best served at room temperature. If made ahead and refrigerated, the salad should sit out a few minutes or be heated a few seconds in the microwave before serving.

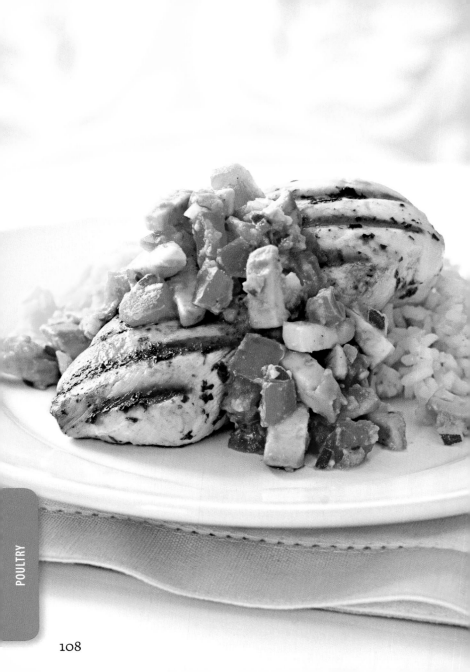

Cilantro-Lime Chicken with Avocado Salsa

A three-minute dip into a pungent marinade is all that's needed to deliver big flavor to chicken breasts. Serve with saffron rice.

- 2 tablespoons minced fresh cilantro
- 2½ tablespoons fresh lime juice
- 1½ tablespoons olive oil
- 4 (6-ounce) skinless, boneless chicken breast halves
- ¼ teaspoon salt
- Cooking spray
- 1 cup chopped plum tomato (about 2)
- 2 tablespoons finely chopped red onion
- 2 teaspoons fresh lime juice
- ¼ teaspoon salt
- ⅛ teaspoon freshly ground black pepper
- 1 avocado, peeled and finely chopped

1. To prepare chicken, combine first 4 ingredients in a large bowl; toss and let stand 3 minutes. Remove chicken from marinade; discard marinade. Sprinkle chicken evenly with ¼ teaspoon salt. Heat a grill pan over medium-high heat. Coat pan with cooking spray. Add chicken to pan; cook 6 minutes on each side or until done. **2.** To prepare salsa, combine tomato and next 4 ingredients in a medium bowl. Add avocado; stir gently to combine. Serve salsa over chicken. **YIELD:** 4 servings (serving size: 1 chicken breast half and about ¼ cup salsa).

CALORIES 289; FAT 13.2g (sat 2.4g, mono 7.5g, poly 1.9g); PROTEIN 35.6g; CARB 6.6g; FIBER 3.6g; CHOL 94mg; IRON 1.6mg; SODIUM 383mg; CALC 29mg

RECIPE BENEFITS: healthy fats; low-sodium

KEY INGREDIENT: Avocados are high in fat, but 64 percent of it is the heart-healthy monounsaturated variety. They also offer other nutrients such as vitamin E, cholesterol-controlling plant sterols, and potassium.

Sauté Skinless, Boneless Chicken Breasts

"Sauté" is a French term that refers to cooking food quickly in a hot pan in a small amount of fat. Skinless, boneless chicken breast halves are great candidates for this cooking method.

- 2 tablespoons extra-virgin olive oil
- 4 (6-ounce) skinless, boneless chicken breast halves
- ½ teaspoon kosher salt
- ½ teaspoon freshly ground black pepper

1. Heat oil in a large skillet over medium-high heat. Sprinkle chicken evenly on both sides with salt and pepper. Add chicken to pan; cook 4 minutes on each side or until golden brown and done. **Yield:** 4 servings (serving size: 1 chicken breast half).

CALORIES 202; FAT 9.8g (sat 1.8g, mono 6g, poly 1.4g); PROTEIN 26.7g; CARB 0.2g; FIBER 0.1g; CHOL 73mg; IRON 1mg; SODIUM 359mg; CALC 14mg

DRESS UP CHICKEN BREASTS WITH PAN SAUCES

WHITE WINE SAUCE: Heat a skillet over medium-high heat. Coat pan with cooking spray. Add ⅓ cup finely chopped onion to pan; sauté 2 minutes, stirring frequently. Stir in ½ cup fat-free, less-sodium chicken broth; ¼ cup dry white wine; and 2 tablespoons white wine vinegar. Bring to a boil. Cook until reduced to ¼ cup (about 5 minutes). Remove from heat; stir in 2 tablespoons butter and 2 teaspoons finely chopped fresh chives. **Yield:** 6 tablespoons (serving size: 1½ tablespoons).

CALORIES 59; FAT 5.7g (sat 3.6g, mono 1.5g, poly 0.2g); PROTEIN 0.6g; CARB 1.6g; FIBER 0.4g; CHOL 15mg; IRON 0.2mg; SODIUM 90mg; CALC 8mg

SPICY ORANGE SAUCE: Heat a skillet over medium-high heat; coat with cooking spray. Add 1 tablespoon grated ginger; sauté 1 minute, stirring constantly. Stir in $\frac{2}{3}$ cup fat-free, less-sodium chicken broth, 3 tablespoons orange marmalade, and $1\frac{1}{2}$ tablespoons low-sodium soy sauce; bring to a boil. Cook until mixture is slightly thick. Stir in $1\frac{1}{2}$ teaspoons fresh lemon juice and $\frac{3}{4}$ teaspoon sambal oelek (or other hot chile sauce). **Yield:** about $\frac{3}{4}$ cup (serving size: about 3 tablespoons).

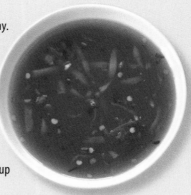

CALORIES 45; FAT 0.1g (sat 0g, mono 0.1g, poly 0g); PROTEIN 0.8g; CARB 11.2g; FIBER 0.4g; CHOL 0mg; IRON 0.2mg; SODIUM 273mg; CALC 10mg

TANGY MUSTARD SAUCE: Heat 2 teaspoons olive oil in a skillet over medium-high heat. Add 2 minced garlic cloves to pan; sauté 30 seconds, stirring constantly. Stir in $\frac{1}{4}$ cup dry white wine, $\frac{1}{4}$ cup fat-free, less-sodium chicken broth, 2 tablespoons maple syrup, and 2 tablespoons Dijon mustard; bring to a boil. Cook until reduced to $\frac{1}{4}$ cup (about 5 minutes), stirring occasionally. Stir in $\frac{3}{4}$ teaspoon chopped fresh rosemary and $\frac{1}{2}$ teaspoon freshly ground black pepper. **Yield:** $\frac{1}{4}$ cup (serving size: 1 tablespoon).

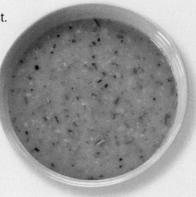

CALORIES 54; FAT 2.3g (sat 0.3g, mono 1.7g, poly 0.3g); PROTEIN 0.3g; CARB 8.2g; FIBER 0.2g; CHOL 0mg; IRON 0.3mg; SODIUM 87mg; CALC 13mg

Scaloppine are chicken breasts pounded thin; they cook to perfection in four minutes. The crisp salad comes together quickly, too, which makes this a great dinner for a busy night.

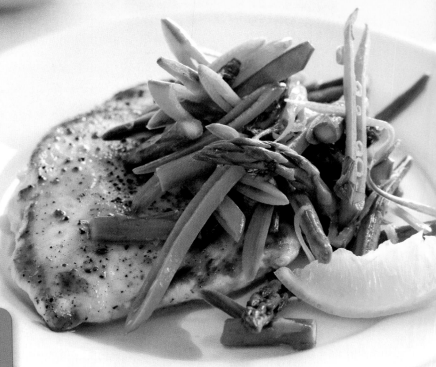

Chicken Scaloppine with Sugar Snap Pea, Asparagus, and Lemon Salad

3 cups julienne-cut trimmed sugar snap peas (about 1 pound)

2 cups (1-inch) sliced asparagus (about 1 pound)

6 (6-ounce) skinless, boneless chicken breast halves

¾ teaspoon salt, divided

½ teaspoon freshly ground black pepper

Cooking spray

1 cup fat-free, less-sodium chicken broth

⅓ cup dry white wine

1 tablespoon butter

1 tablespoon chopped fresh mint

2½ tablespoons extra-virgin olive oil

1 teaspoon grated lemon rind

1½ tablespoons fresh lemon juice

6 lemon wedges

1. Steam peas and asparagus, covered, 4 minutes or until crisp-tender. Rinse pea mixture with cold water; drain. Chill.

2. Place each chicken breast half between 2 sheets of heavy-duty plastic wrap; pound to ¼-inch thickness using a meat mallet or small heavy skillet. Sprinkle chicken evenly with ½ teaspoon salt and pepper. Heat a large nonstick skillet over medium-high heat. Coat pan with cooking spray. Add 2 breast halves to pan; sauté 2 minutes on each side or until done. Repeat procedure twice with remaining chicken. Add broth and wine to pan; bring to a boil, scraping pan to loosen browned bits. Cook until reduced to ½ cup (about 5 minutes). Remove from heat; stir in butter.

3. Combine remaining ¼ teaspoon salt, mint, oil, rind, and juice, stirring well with a whisk. Drizzle oil mixture over pea mixture; toss gently to coat. Serve pea mixture with chicken and sauce. Garnish with lemon wedges. **YIELD:** 6 servings (serving size: 1 chicken breast half, about 1 cup pea mixture, 4 teaspoons sauce, and 1 lemon wedge).

CALORIES 315; FAT 10g (sat 2.6g, mono 5.2g, poly 1.4g); PROTEIN 43.3g; CARB 10.3g; FIBER 3.7g; CHOL 104mg; IRON 4.1mg; SODIUM 495mg; CALC 98mg

Peanut-Crusted Chicken with Pineapple Salsa

Pick up a container of fresh pineapple chunks in the produce section of the supermarket; chop into half-inch pieces for the salsa. Serve with steamed broccoli and warm rolls to complete the dinner.

1 cup chopped fresh pineapple
2 tablespoons chopped fresh cilantro
1 tablespoon finely chopped red onion
$^1/_3$ cup unsalted, dry-roasted peanuts
1 (1-ounce) slice white bread
$^1/_2$ teaspoon salt
$^1/_8$ teaspoon black pepper
4 (4-ounce) chicken cutlets
$1^1/_2$ teaspoons canola oil
Cooking spray
Cilantro sprigs (optional)

1. Combine first 3 ingredients in a small bowl, tossing well.
2. Place peanuts and bread slice in a food processor; process until finely chopped. Sprinkle salt and pepper evenly over chicken. Dredge chicken in breadcrumb mixture.
3. Heat oil in a large nonstick skillet coated with cooking spray over medium-high heat. Add chicken to pan; cook 2 minutes on each side or until done. Serve chicken with pineapple mixture. Garnish with cilantro sprigs, if desired. YIELD: 4 servings (serving size: 1 cutlet and $^1/_4$ cup salsa).

CALORIES 219; FAT 7.4g (sat 1.1g, mono 3.4g, poly 2.1g); PROTEIN 28.9g; CARB 9.1g; FIBER 1.3g; CHOL 66mg; IRON 1.2mg; SODIUM 398mg; CALC 27mg

RECIPE BENEFIT: healthy fats

POULTRY

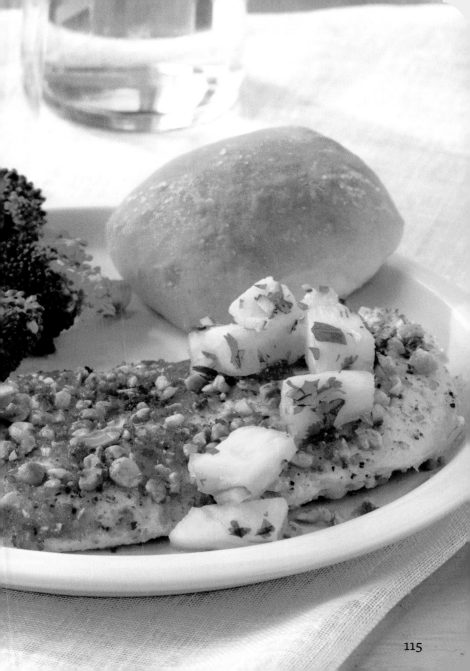

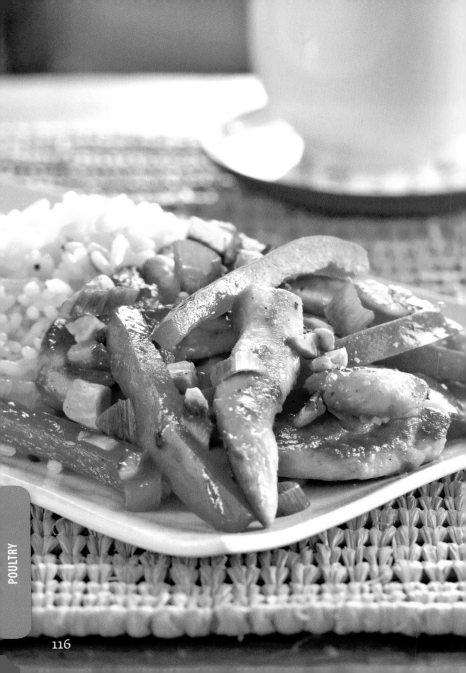

Chicken, Cashew, and Red Pepper Stir-Fry

This dish balances salty, sweet, tangy, and spicy ingredients.
Spoon it alongside cooked jasmine or basmati rice.

3¾ teaspoons cornstarch, divided
2 tablespoons low-sodium soy sauce, divided
2 teaspoons dry sherry
1 teaspoon rice wine vinegar
¾ teaspoon sugar
½ teaspoon hot pepper sauce (such as Tabasco)
1 pound chicken breast tenders, cut lengthwise into thin strips
½ cup coarsely chopped unsalted cashews
2 tablespoons canola oil
2 cups julienne-cut red bell pepper (about 1 large)
1 teaspoon minced garlic
½ teaspoon minced peeled fresh ginger
3 tablespoons thinly sliced green onions

1. Combine 1 teaspoon cornstarch, 1 tablespoon soy sauce, and next 4 ingredients in a small bowl; stir with a whisk.

2. Combine remaining 2¾ teaspoons cornstarch, remaining 1 tablespoon soy sauce, and chicken in a medium bowl; toss well to coat.

3. Heat a large nonstick skillet over medium-high heat. Add cashews to pan; cook 3 minutes or until lightly toasted, stirring frequently. Remove from pan.

4. Add oil to pan, swirling to coat. Add chicken mixture to pan; sauté 2 minutes or until lightly browned. Remove chicken from pan; place in a bowl. Add bell pepper to pan; sauté 2 minutes, stirring occasionally. Add garlic and ginger; cook 30 seconds. Add chicken and cornstarch mixture to pan; cook 1 minute or until sauce is slightly thick. Sprinkle with cashews and green onions. **YIELD:** 4 servings (serving size: 1 cup).

CALORIES 324; FAT 16.6g (sat 2.5g, mono 9.2g, poly 3.8g); PROTEIN 30g; CARB 13.5g; FIBER 2g; CHOL 66mg; IRON 2.4mg; SODIUM 350mg; CALC 33mg

Although the tomato mixture and tangy lemon marinade complement the flavorful chicken thighs, you can use this same preparation with tuna steaks. Roast the tomatoes while the chicken marinates. Garnish with fresh parsley.

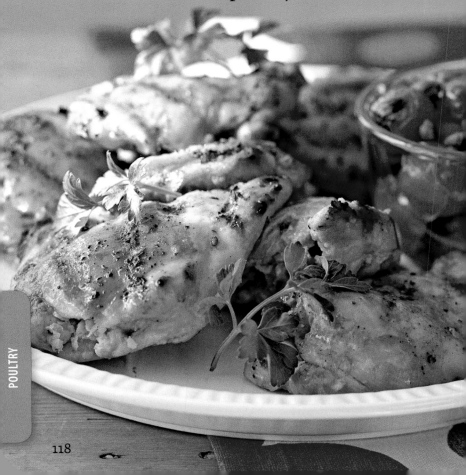

Grilled Chicken Thighs with Roasted Grape Tomatoes

1 tablespoon grated lemon rind
2 tablespoons fresh lemon juice
1 teaspoon olive oil
2 garlic cloves, minced
8 skinless, boneless chicken thighs (about $1^{1}/_{2}$ pounds)
$^{1}/_{2}$ teaspoon salt
$^{1}/_{4}$ teaspoon freshly ground black pepper
Cooking spray

2 cups grape tomatoes
2 teaspoons olive oil
2 tablespoons chopped fresh parsley
1 teaspoon grated lemon rind
1 tablespoon fresh lemon juice
1 tablespoon capers
$^{1}/_{8}$ teaspoon salt
$^{1}/_{8}$ teaspoon freshly ground black pepper

1. Prepare grill.

2. To prepare chicken, combine first 4 ingredients in a large zip-top plastic bag. Add chicken to bag; seal. Marinate in refrigerator 15 minutes, turning bag occasionally.

3. Remove chicken from bag; discard marinade. Sprinkle chicken evenly with $^{1}/_{2}$ teaspoon salt and $^{1}/_{4}$ teaspoon pepper. Place chicken on grill rack coated with cooking spray; grill 5 minutes on each side or until done.

4. Preheat oven to 425°.

5. To prepare tomatoes, combine tomatoes and 2 teaspoons oil in an 8-inch square baking dish; toss gently. Bake at 425° for 18 minutes or until tomatoes are tender. Combine tomato mixture, parsley, and remaining ingredients, stirring gently. Serve with chicken. YIELD: 4 servings (serving size: 2 chicken thighs and $^{1}/_{4}$ cup tomato mixture).

CALORIES 194; FAT 7.8g (sat 1.7g, mono 3.4g, poly 1.6g); PROTEIN 25.9g; CARB 4.5g; FIBER 1.1g; CHOL 106mg; IRON 1.9mg; SODIUM 329mg; CALC 23mg

Chicken Bulgur Salad

Reminiscent of tabbouleh, this Lebanese-inspired dish is a smart choice if you want to incorporate more fiber into your diet. Bulgur—wheat berries that have been steamed, dried, and ground—is the basis of many salads in the Middle East. Serve this salad with warmed whole-wheat pita bread.

- 1 **cup water**
- ½ **cup uncooked quick-cooking bulgur**
- 1½ **cups cubed cooked chicken breast (about ½ pound)**
- 1 **cup finely chopped fresh parsley**
- 1 **(14-ounce) can quartered artichoke hearts, drained and coarsely chopped**
- 1 **cup grape tomatoes, halved**
- ⅓ **cup light Northern Italian salad dressing with basil and Romano (such as Ken's Steak House Lite)**
- 2 **tablespoons fresh lemon juice**

1. Bring 1 cup water to a boil in a medium saucepan; stir in bulgur. Return to a boil; reduce heat, cover, and simmer 8 minutes or until liquid is absorbed. Drain bulgur, and rinse with cold water; drain well.

2. Combine chicken and remaining ingredients in a large bowl, tossing to coat. Add bulgur; toss gently to coat. **YIELD:** 4 servings (serving size: 1¼ cups).

CALORIES 228; FAT 6g (sat 1g, mono 1g, poly 0.5g); PROTEIN 21.2g; CARB 22.8g; FIBER 4.5g; CHOL 45mg; IRON 3mg; SODIUM 435mg; CALC 56mg

RECIPE BENEFIT: low-fat

POULTRY

CHOICE INGREDIENT: *Parsley*

No refrigerator should be without parsley. It's the workhorse of the herb world and can go in just about every dish you cook. Parsley's mild, grassy taste doesn't overpower the other ingredients. Flat-leaf parsley is preferred for cooking because it stands up better to heat and has more flavor, while the more decorative curly parsley is used mostly for garnishing.

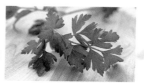

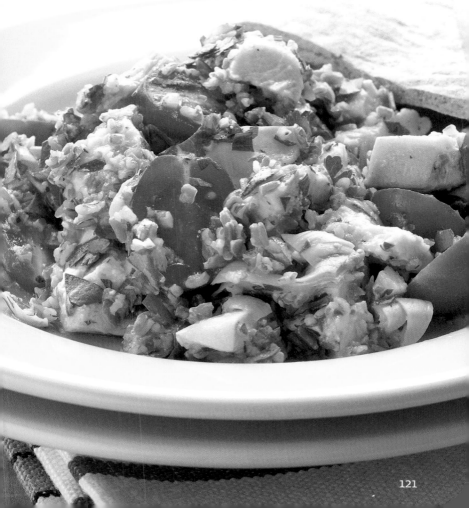

121

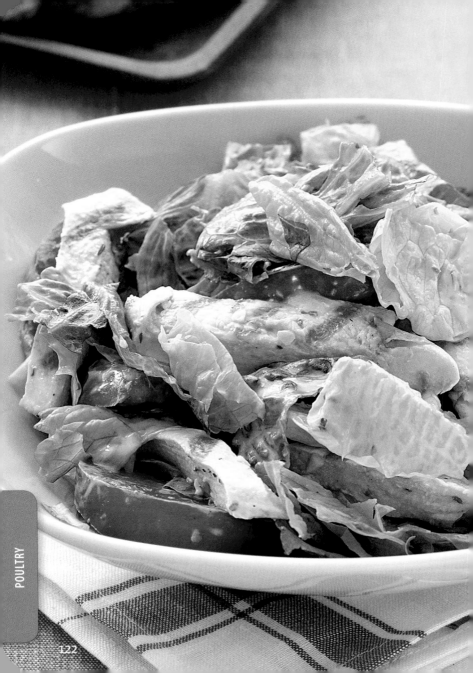

Chicken Caesar Salad

For an easy addition to this salad, place baguette slices on the grill while you're cooking the chicken. Grill the bread slices for 2 minutes on each side; then rub the slices with the cut side of a halved garlic clove.

6 tablespoons light mayonnaise
3 tablespoons fresh lemon juice
1½ tablespoons water
1½ teaspoons anchovy paste
3 large garlic cloves, minced
1 teaspoon dried oregano
½ teaspoon freshly ground black pepper

3 (4-ounce) chicken cutlets
Cooking spray
1 (10-ounce) package romaine salad
2 tomatoes, cut into wedges
¼ cup (1 ounce) grated fresh Parmesan cheese

1. Prepare grill to medium-high heat.

2. While grill heats, combine mayonnaise, lemon juice, and next 5 ingredients in a small bowl, stirring well with a whisk. Reserve ⅓ cup dressing in a separate bowl; set aside.

3. Place chicken on grill rack coated with cooking spray. Grill 2 to 3 minutes on each side or until done, basting frequently with remaining dressing. Remove from grill. Cool slightly; slice.

4. Combine chicken, reserved ⅓ cup dressing, lettuce, and tomato in a large bowl; toss gently to coat. Divide salad among each of 4 bowls. Sprinkle each serving with 1 tablespoon cheese. **YIELD:** 4 servings (serving size: 2½ cups).

CALORIES 225; FAT 11g (sat 2.4g, mono 0.7g, poly 0.4g); PROTEIN 23.6g; CARB 9g; FIBER 2.6g; CHOL 68mg; IRON 1.8mg; SODIUM 446mg; CALC 114mg

Smart Bread Choices

Choose whole grains, and watch portion sizes.

Whole-grain health benefits:

When combined with an overall healthy diet, the dietary fiber found in whole grains reduces blood cholesterol levels and protects against heart disease. According to the American Heart Association, eating the right amount is what really counts. A good rule of thumb to follow is to make at least half of all the grains eaten on a daily basis whole grains.

How to tell if a bread is whole grain:

• Look for "100% whole grain" or "100% whole wheat" on the package. If one of those isn't there, check the ingredient list. The first ingredient should be "whole-wheat flour," "whole grain," "whole oats," or "whole rye" instead of "enriched."

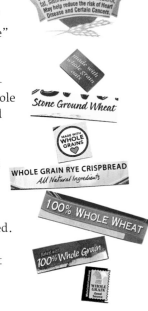

• Look for the Food and Drug Administration–approved claim. It links consumption of whole grains to a reduced risk of heart disease and some types of cancer.

• Look for the black-and-yellow Whole Grain Stamp. The stamp, developed by the Whole Grains Council, guarantees you get at least half a serving (8 grams) of whole grains in each serving—the exact amount will be listed. The stamp can be placed anywhere on the package. This is a voluntary program, so not all whole-grain products carry it.

What is a serving of bread?

Since some large breads—such as hoagies, bagels, and sandwich rolls—can be equal to 4 or 5 servings of grains, make sure you know what's a proper portion size to keep your calories in check. Use the examples below to guide you to the breads that only count as 1 or 2 servings.

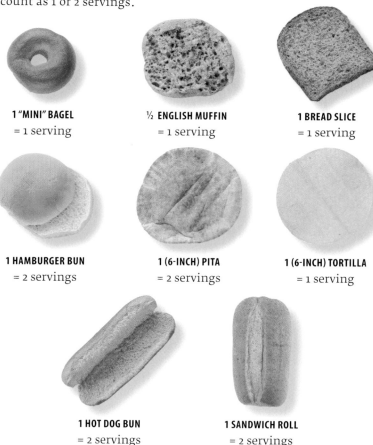

1 "MINI" BAGEL
= 1 serving

½ ENGLISH MUFFIN
= 1 serving

1 BREAD SLICE
= 1 serving

1 HAMBURGER BUN
= 2 servings

1 (6-INCH) PITA
= 2 servings

1 (6-INCH) TORTILLA
= 1 serving

1 HOT DOG BUN
= 2 servings

1 SANDWICH ROLL
= 2 servings

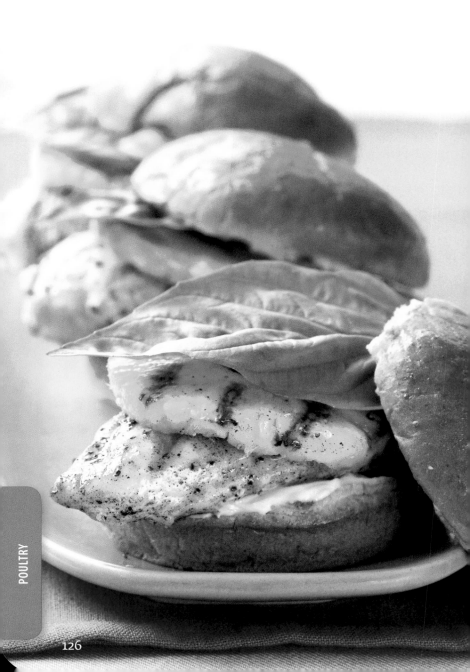

Grilled Chicken and Pineapple Sandwiches

Tickle your palate with a taste of the tropics. Pineapple has a natural juiciness that gives this sandwich an irresistible taste. The fruit also offers a healthy reason for indulging: It's a high source of vitamin C.

4   (6-ounce) skinless, boneless chicken breast halves
½   teaspoon salt
¼   teaspoon freshly ground black pepper
Cooking spray
¼   cup fresh lime juice (about 2 limes)
4   (½-inch-thick) slices fresh pineapple
Light mayonnaise (optional)
4   (1.5-ounce) whole-wheat hamburger buns, toasted
4   large fresh basil leaves

1. Prepare grill.
2. Sprinkle chicken evenly with salt and pepper. Place chicken on grill rack coated with cooking spray; grill 5 to 6 minutes on each side or until done, brushing occasionally with lime juice. Grill pineapple 2 to 3 minutes on each side or until browned.
3. Spread mayonnaise on bottom halves of buns, if desired. Top each with 1 chicken breast half, 1 pineapple slice, 1 basil leaf, and 1 bun top. Serve immediately. YIELD: 4 servings (serving size: 1 sandwich).

CALORIES 333; FAT 4g (sat 0.9g, mono 1g, poly 1.4g); PROTEIN 43.4g; CARB 30.5g; FIBER 4.1g; CHOL 99mg; IRON 2.5mg; SODIUM 608mg; CALC 75mg

RECIPE BENEFIT: low-fat

Mediterranean Turkey Burgers

Prepare a spicy and creamy tzatziki sauce to spread on the burgers or to serve on the side for dipping. Combine $1/2$ cup plain low-fat, Greek-style yogurt; $1/4$ cup finely chopped seeded cucumber; $1/4$ teaspoon salt; and $1/8$ teaspoon ground red pepper. Serve with sliced bell pepper and celery sticks.

$1/2$ cup panko (Japanese breadcrumbs)
$1/4$ cup (1 ounce) crumbled feta cheese
1 tablespoon minced red onion
2 tablespoons commercial pesto
$1/4$ teaspoon salt
$1/4$ teaspoon freshly ground black pepper

1 pound ground turkey breast
1 garlic clove, minced
Cooking spray
2 cups arugula
2 (6-inch) whole-wheat pitas, toasted and halved

1. Combine first 8 ingredients in a bowl; mix until combined. Divide panko mixture into 4 portions, shaping each into a $1/2$-inch-thick oval patty.

2. Heat a nonstick grill pan over medium-high heat. Coat pan with cooking spray. Add patties to pan; cook 6 minutes on each side or until done. Place 1 patty and $1/2$ cup arugula in each pita half. **YIELD:** 4 servings (serving size: 1 stuffed pita half).

CALORIES 303; FAT 8.8g (sat 2.9g, mono 4.1g, poly 0.8g); PROTEIN 33g; CARB 24.3g; FIBER 3g; CHOL 56mg; IRON 1.9mg; SODIUM 595mg; CALC 101mg

RECIPE BENEFIT: low-fat

POULTRY

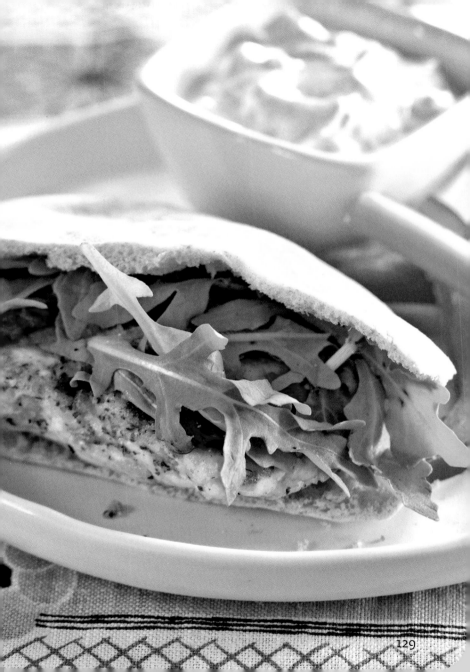

Broths & Stocks

Broths and stocks seem simple, but ingredient labels can reveal lots of sodium, frequent use of protein additives, and vague flavorings.

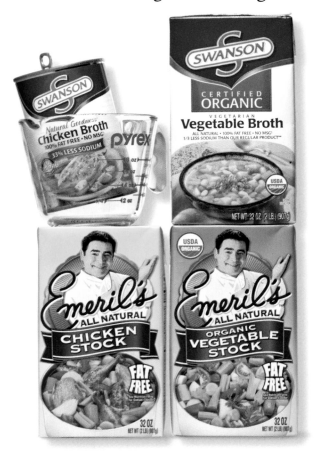

What to look for:

Purchased broths and stocks can harbor lots of sodium, so read the label and choose one that contains 700 milligrams of sodium or less per cup. Be aware that some broths and stocks meet this criteria but aren't labeled "low-sodium" or "less-sodium." You should also know that the term "less-sodium" doesn't mean it's low in sodium—it means the product contains less sodium than the original.

FAVORITE CHICKEN: SWANSON® LESS-SODIUM, FAT-FREE CHICKEN BROTH

This broth has a pleasant roast chicken flavor and aroma, and at $3 per 32-ounce carton, it won't break the bank either. This is our Test Kitchens' go-to option for recipes.

FAVORITE VEGETABLE: SWANSON® CERTIFIED ORGANIC VEGETABLE BROTH

This broth has a richness and butteriness with a balance of celery, onion, and carrot.

GOOD CHICKEN: EMERIL'S® ALL NATURAL CHICKEN STOCK

The less-pronounced chicken essence in this stock is balanced with plenty of aromatics. It also has a pleasant saltiness. Though not labeled low-sodium, the sodium count is similar to that of the Swanson low-sodium chicken broth.

GOOD VEGETABLE: EMERIL'S® ALL NATURAL ORGANIC VEGETABLE STOCK

This broth has a neutral flavor with a slightly sweet aftertaste that makes it a good stock or broth choice.

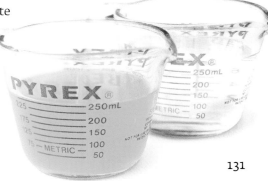

Chicken-Escarole Soup

To cut down on time and keep cleanup to a minimum, use kitchen shears to easily chop tomatoes while they're still in the can.

1 (14½-ounce) can Italian-style stewed tomatoes, undrained and chopped

1 (14-ounce) can fat-free, less-sodium chicken broth

1 cup chopped cooked chicken breast

2 cups coarsely chopped escarole (about 1 small head)

2 teaspoons extra-virgin olive oil

1. Combine tomatoes and broth in a large saucepan. Cover and bring to a boil over high heat. Reduce heat to low; simmer 5 minutes. Add chicken, escarole, and oil; cook 5 minutes. **YIELD:** 4 servings (serving size: 1 cup).

CALORIES 118; FAT 4g (sat 0.7g, mono 2.1g, poly 0.6g); PROTEIN 13.5g; CARB 7.9g; FIBER 1.5g; CHOL 30mg; IRON 1.1mg; SODIUM 535mg; CALC 49mg

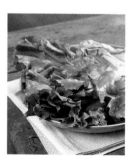

CHOICE INGREDIENT: Escarole, a variety of endive, is not as bitter as Belgian endive or curly endive. It has broad, bright green leaves that grow in loose heads. When purchasing escarole, look for fresh, crisp leaves without discoloration. Store escarole tightly wrapped in the refrigerator for up to three days.

POULTRY

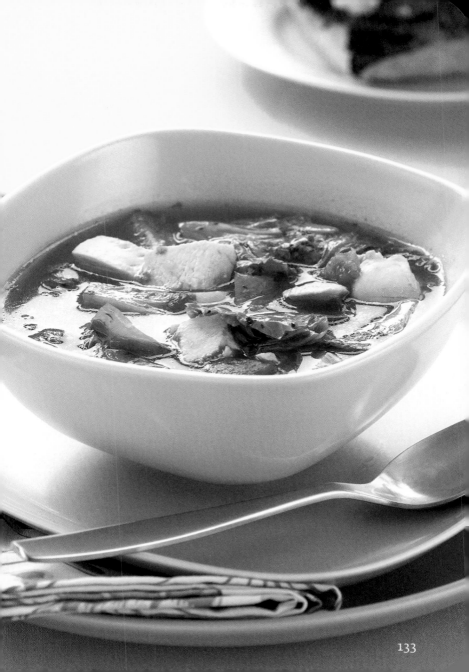

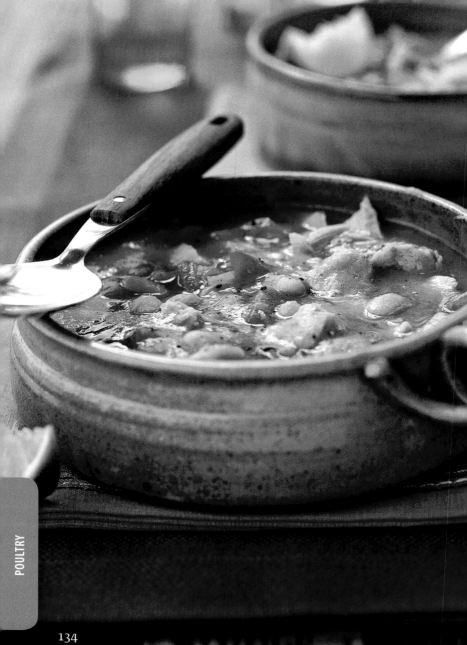

White Bean and Turkey Chili

Using canned beans and chicken broth make this crowd-pleasing chili convenient.

1 tablespoon canola oil	3 cups chopped cooked turkey
2 cups diced yellow onion (about 2 medium)	1/2 cup diced seeded plum tomato (about 1)
1 1/2 tablespoons chili powder	1/3 cup chopped fresh cilantro
1 tablespoon minced garlic	2 tablespoons fresh lime juice
1 1/2 teaspoons ground cumin	1/2 teaspoon salt
1 teaspoon dried oregano	1/2 teaspoon freshly ground black pepper
3 (15.8-ounce) cans Great Northern beans, rinsed and drained	8 lime wedges (optional)
4 cups fat-free, less-sodium chicken broth	

1. Heat oil in a large Dutch oven over medium-high heat. Add onion; sauté 10 minutes or until tender and golden. Add chili powder, garlic, and cumin; sauté 2 minutes. Add oregano and beans; cook 30 seconds. Add broth; bring to a simmer. Cook 20 minutes.

2. Place 2 cups of bean mixture in a blender or food processor, and process until smooth. Return pureed mixture to pan. Add turkey, and cook 5 minutes or until thoroughly heated. Remove from heat. Add diced tomato, chopped cilantro, lime juice, salt, and pepper, stirring well. Garnish with lime wedges, if desired.

YIELD: 8 servings (serving size: about 1 cup).

CALORIES 286; FAT 6g (sat 1.2g, mono 2.1g, poly 1.6g); PROTEIN 32.4g; CARB 24.3g; FIBER 5.5g; CHOL 85mg; IRON 4.8mg; SODIUM 435mg; CALC 105mg

RECIPE BENEFITS: low-fat; high-fiber

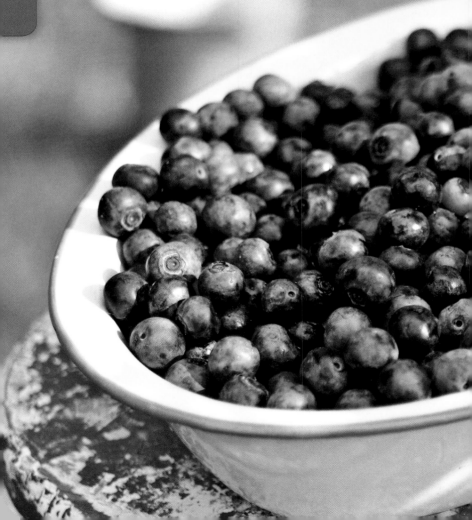

HEALTHY HEART
Desserts

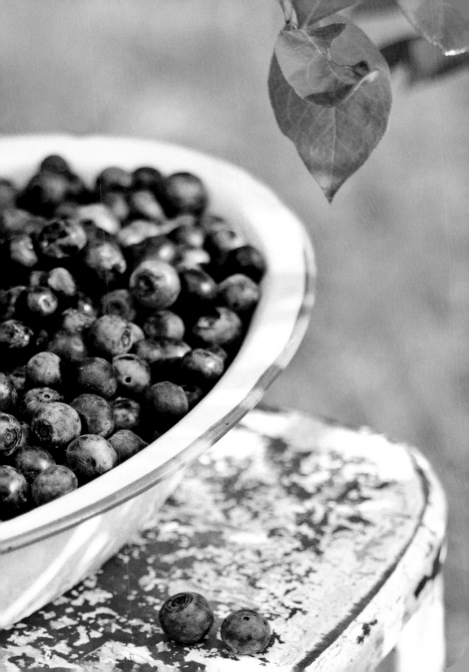

Chocolate

Mounting evidence shows that certain forms of chocolate may be good for your health. The key is in the cocoa content.

What to look for:

When the right kind is eaten in moderation, chocolate may help reduce high blood pressure, reduce LDL (the "bad cholesterol"), or even provide potential cancer-fighting benefits. Chocolate and cocoa come from a plant—the cacao (pronounced ca-COW)—and contain plant compounds that researchers credit with these health benefits. However, researchers don't attribute these effects to milk chocolate bars or chocolate-coated candies but specifically to dark chocolate and minimally processed cocoa powder—the more cocoa in the chocolate, the more antioxidants it contains. You'll want to avoid highly alkalized, or Dutch process, as this can significantly reduce the beneficial compounds found in chocolate. Choose dark chocolate with a cocoa content of 70% or more, and limit your portion to about 1.5 ounces. That ensures you'll reap the health benefits without adding too many calories.

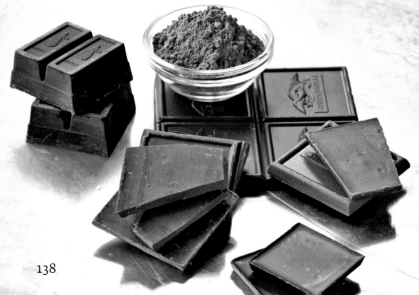

Cookies, Brownies & Snack Cakes

Be sure to check the label on these premade baked sweet treats—they're often among the prime places trans fats are found in the grocery store.

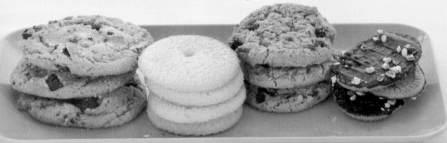

What to look for:

Like most desserts, packaged cookies, brownies, and snack cakes can be high in saturated fat, sugars, and calories per serving, so moderation is key. If you eat these products regularly, watch out for those loaded with sugar, and choose those that contain 10 grams or less per serving and preferably as little saturated fat as possible—no more than 1 gram per serving.

Watch out for trans fats.

Individually wrapped and premade desserts can be a jackpot for trans fats—one serving can contain more than the daily maximum amount of trans fats that the American Heart Association considers safe. The same goes for the treats found in the grocery store bakery. For both, you should make sure the ingredient list doesn't include partially hydrogenated oils. Organic products and those made with all-natural ingredients are usually the best bets. Better yet, make your own from scratch.

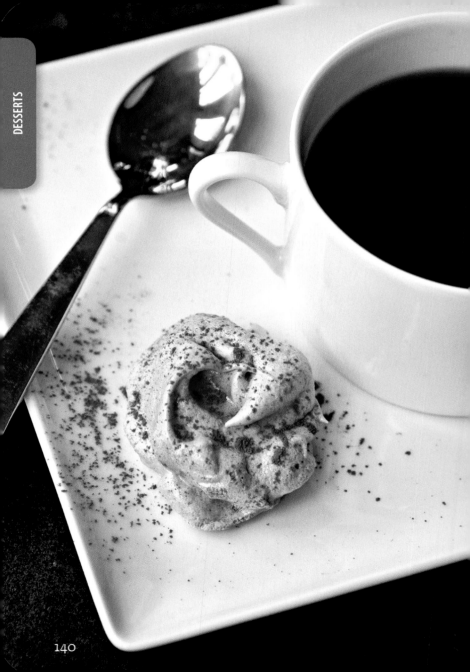

Cocoa Nib Meringues

Superfine sugar dissolves easily into the meringue for a supple texture. If you can't find superfine sugar, process granulated sugar in a blender for a minute or two. Store meringues in an airtight container for up to one day.

- $1/2$ teaspoon cream of tartar
- 3 large egg whites
- $1/2$ cup superfine sugar
- 2 tablespoons unsweetened cocoa
- 2 teaspoons cocoa nibs
- 1 teaspoon instant espresso granules or 2 teaspoons instant coffee granules
- Dash of salt
- 1 teaspoon unsweetened cocoa (optional)

1. Preheat oven to 225°.

2. Line a baking sheet with parchment paper.

3. Place cream of tartar and egg whites in a large bowl; beat with a mixer at high speed until foamy. Gradually add superfine sugar, 1 tablespoon at a time, beating until stiff peaks form. Add 2 tablespoons unsweetened cocoa, cocoa nibs, instant espresso granules, and salt; beat just until blended.

4. Drop batter by level tablespoons onto prepared baking sheet. Bake at 225° for 1 hour. Turn oven off (do not remove pan from oven); cool meringues in closed oven at least 8 hours or until crisp. Carefully remove meringues from paper. Sprinkle with 1 teaspoon unsweetened cocoa, if desired. **YIELD:** 36 meringues (serving size: 1 meringue).

CALORIES 14; FAT 0.1g (sat 0.1g, mono 0g, poly 0g); PROTEIN 0.4g; CARB 3.1g; FIBER 0.1g; CHOL 0mg; IRON 0.1mg; SODIUM 9mg; CALC 1mg

RECIPE BENEFIT: fat-free

Brownie Bites

Cocoa nibs, which are broken bits of husked cocoa beans, add delicate chocolate flavor and delicious nutty crunch to baked goods. You can find cocoa nibs at upscale supermarkets and gourmet cookware stores. When you make this recipe, don't be alarmed that the batter is very wet—the end result will be moist, tender minicakes.

2.25 ounces self-rising flour (about $^1/_2$ cup)
$^2/_3$ cup sugar
3 tablespoons unsweetened cocoa
4 large egg whites
2 tablespoons canola oil
3 tablespoons chocolate liqueur (optional)

$^1/_3$ cup cocoa nibs
Cooking spray
Roasted salted almonds (such as Blue Diamond), coarsely chopped (optional)
Powdered sugar (optional)

1. Preheat oven to 400°.

2. Weigh or lightly spoon flour into a dry measuring cup; level with a knife. Combine flour, sugar, and cocoa in a medium bowl, stirring with a whisk.

3. Whisk egg whites until foamy in a separate bowl. Add oil and liqueur, if desired, stirring with a whisk. Add egg white mixture to flour mixture, stirring just until moistened. Fold in cocoa nibs. Spoon batter evenly into 24 miniature muffin cups coated with cooking spray. Sprinkle batter evenly with almonds, if desired.

4. Bake at 400° for 8 minutes. Remove from pans; cool on wire racks. Sprinkle with powdered sugar, if desired. **YIELD:** 24 servings (serving size: 1 brownie bite).

CALORIES 61; FAT 2.4g (sat 0.8g, mono 0.9g, poly 0.4g); PROTEIN 1.2g; CARB 8.8g; FIBER 0.3g; CHOL 0mg; IRON 0.4mg; SODIUM 43mg; CALC 15mg

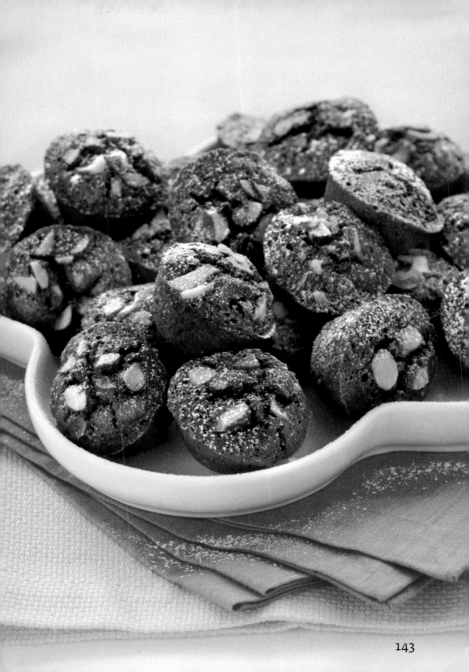

Chocolate Lava Cakes with Pistachio Cream

1 cup shelled dry-roasted
  pistachios
1³/₄ cups sugar, divided
 ¹/₄ cup unsweetened cocoa
  2 large eggs
  5 large egg whites
  2 ounces bittersweet chocolate,
    coarsely chopped

 ¹/₂ teaspoon baking powder
 ¹/₂ teaspoon vanilla extract
Cooking spray
  1 cup 2% reduced-fat milk
Dash of salt
Powdered sugar (optional)

1. Place pistachios in a food processor; process until a crumbly paste forms (about 3¹/₂ minutes), scraping sides of bowl once.

2. Place ¹/₄ cup pistachio butter, 1¹/₄ cups sugar, cocoa, eggs, and egg whites in top of a double boiler; stir well with a whisk. Add chocolate; cook over simmering water until chocolate melts and sugar dissolves (about 3 minutes). Remove from heat; add baking powder and vanilla. Stir with a whisk until smooth. Spoon batter into 12 muffin cups coated with cooking spray. Chill 2 hours.

3. Place remaining ¹/₄ cup pistachio butter and ¹/₂ cup sugar in food processor; pulse 4 times or until combined. Add milk and salt; process until smooth. Strain mixture through a sieve into a small saucepan; discard solids. Bring to a boil. Reduce heat; simmer 4 minutes or until thick. Remove from heat; pour into a bowl. Cover and chill.

4. Preheat oven to 450°.

5. Bake cakes at 450° for 9 minutes or until almost set (centers will not be firm). Let cool in pan 5 minutes. Invert each cake onto a dessert plate; drizzle with sauce. Garnish with powdered sugar, if desired. **YIELD:** 12 servings (serving size: 1 cake and 2 teaspoons sauce).

CALORIES 232; FAT 7.7g (sat 2.2g, mono 3.1g, poly 1.5g); PROTEIN 6.1g; CARB 37.2g; FIBER 2g; CHOL 37mg; IRON 0.9mg; SODIUM 73mg; CALC 51mg

These flourless chocolate cakes are as rich as a restaurant dessert, but they're made with a fraction of the fat and no butter. When these cakes bake, the gooey filling causes the center to sink in.

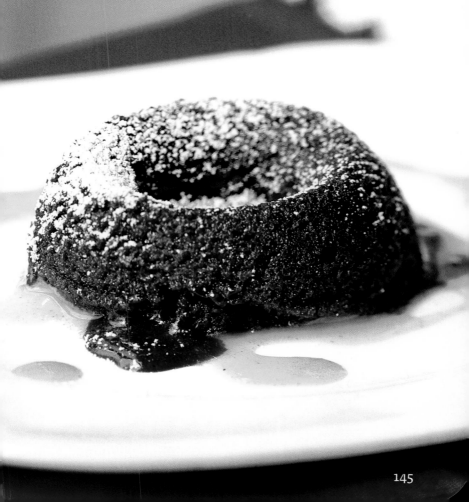

take two:

Homemade vs. Oven-Ready
chocolate chip cookies

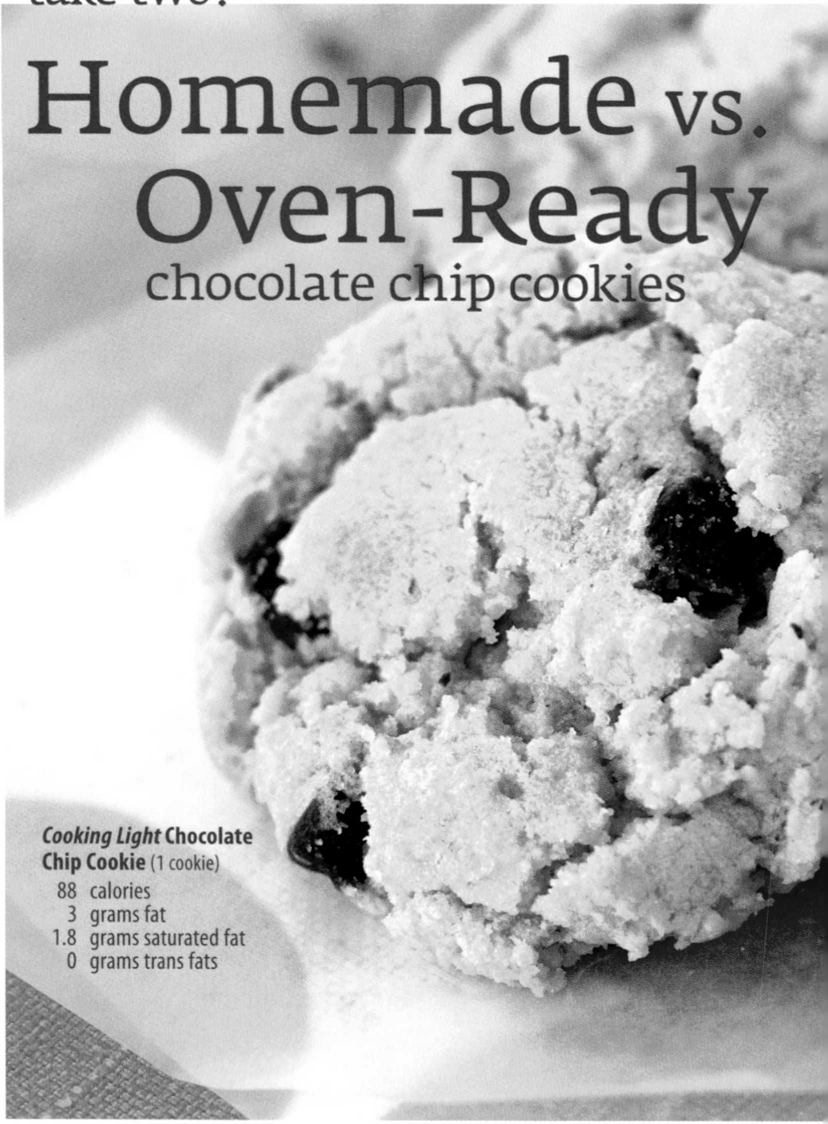

***Cooking Light* Chocolate Chip Cookie** (1 cookie)

- 88 calories
- 3 grams fat
- 1.8 grams saturated fat
- 0 grams trans fats

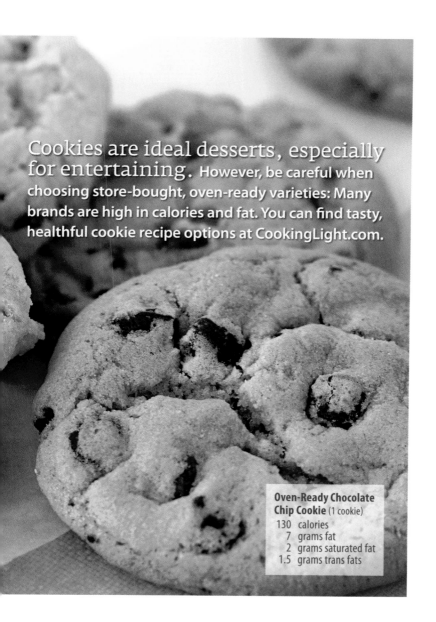

Cookies are ideal desserts, especially for entertaining. However, be careful when choosing store-bought, oven-ready varieties: Many brands are high in calories and fat. You can find tasty, healthful cookie recipe options at CookingLight.com.

Oven-Ready Chocolate Chip Cookie (1 cookie)

130	calories
7	grams fat
2	grams saturated fat
1.5	grams trans fats

Cocoa Fudge Cookies

You can mix these incredibly easy, fudgy cookies right in the saucepan. When freshly baked, these thin cookies have crisp edges and chewy centers. You can make them with either Dutch process or natural unsweetened cocoa powder; we opted for the latter.

4.5 ounces all-purpose flour (about 1 cup)
¼ teaspoon baking soda
⅛ teaspoon salt
5 tablespoons butter
7 tablespoons unsweetened cocoa

⅔ cup granulated sugar
⅓ cup packed brown sugar
⅓ cup plain low-fat yogurt
1 teaspoon vanilla extract
Cooking spray

1. Preheat oven to 350°.

2. Weigh or lightly spoon flour into a dry measuring cup; level with a knife. Combine flour, soda, and salt; set aside. Melt butter in a large saucepan over medium heat. Remove from heat; stir in cocoa and sugars (mixture will resemble coarse sand). Add yogurt and vanilla, stirring to combine. Add flour mixture, stirring until moist. Drop by level tablespoons 2 inches apart onto baking sheets coated with cooking spray.

3. Bake at 350° for 8 to 10 minutes or until almost set. Cool on pans 2 to 3 minutes or until firm. Remove cookies from pans; cool on wire racks. **YIELD:** 2 dozen (serving size: 1 cookie).

CALORIES 78; FAT 2.7g (sat 1.6g, mono 0.8g, poly 0.1g); PROTEIN 1g; CARB 13.4g; FIBER 0.5g; CHOL 7mg; IRON 0.5mg; SODIUM 54mg; CALC 12mg

RECIPE BENEFITS: low-fat; low-sodium

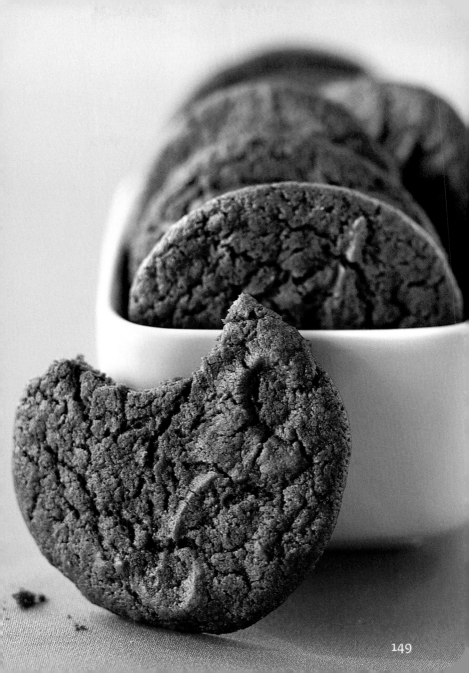

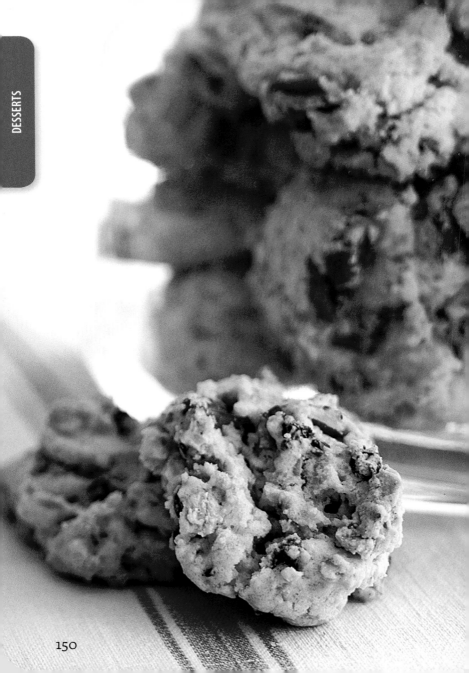

Oatmeal, Chocolate Chip, and Pecan Cookies

These easy drop cookies are crisp on the outside and slightly chewy on the inside. Chocolate minichips disperse better in the batter, but you can use regular chips, if desired.

5.5	ounces all-purpose flour (about 1¼ cups)	½	cup packed brown sugar
1	cup regular oats	⅓	cup butter, softened
¾	teaspoon baking powder	1½	teaspoons vanilla extract
½	teaspoon baking soda	1	large egg
½	teaspoon salt	¼	cup chopped pecans, toasted
¾	cup granulated sugar	¼	cup semisweet chocolate minichips

1. Preheat oven to 350°.

2. Weigh or lightly spoon flour into dry measuring cups; level with a knife. Combine flour and next 4 ingredients, stirring with a whisk; set aside.

3. Place sugars and butter in a large bowl; beat with a mixer at medium speed until well blended. Add vanilla and egg; beat until blended. Gradually add flour mixture, beating at low speed just until combined. Stir in pecans and minichips. Drop dough by level tablespoons 2 inches apart onto baking sheets lined with parchment paper. Bake at 350° for 12 minutes or until edges of cookies are lightly browned. Cool on pans 2 minutes. Remove cookies from pans; cool on wire racks. YIELD: 3 dozen (serving size: 1 cookie).

CALORIES 81; FAT 3g (sat 1.4g, mono 1g, poly 0.3g); PROTEIN 1.1g; CARB 12.9g; FIBER 0.5g; CHOL 10mg; IRON 0.5mg; SODIUM 76mg; CALC 12mg

RECIPE BENEFIT: low-sodium

Oatmeal-Raisin Cookies

Fast, simple, and satisfying, Oatmeal-Raisin Cookies are a sure-to-please staple in the American home. They're easy to prepare because they're made with ingredients that you probably have on hand. Your kitchen will smell flavorful and inviting when you pop a batch in the oven.

$1/2$ cup granulated sugar
$1/2$ cup packed brown sugar
$1/3$ cup butter, softened
1 teaspoon vanilla extract
$1/8$ teaspoon salt
1 large egg

4.5 ounces all-purpose flour (about 1 cup)
1 cup regular oats
$1/2$ cup raisins
Cooking spray

1. Preheat oven to 350°.

2. Beat first 6 ingredients with a mixer at medium speed until light and fluffy. Weigh or lightly spoon flour into a dry measuring cup; level with a knife. Add flour and oats to egg mixture, and beat until blended. Stir in raisins. Drop by level tablespoons 2 inches apart onto baking sheets coated with cooking spray. Bake at 350° for 15 minutes or until golden brown. Cool on pans 3 minutes. Remove cookies from pans; cool on wire racks. **YIELD:** 2 dozen (serving size: 1 cookie).

CALORIES 101; FAT 3.1g (sat 1.7g, mono 0.9g, poly 0.2g); PROTEIN 1.5g; CARB 17.3g; FIBER 0.6g; CHOL 16mg; IRON 0.6mg; SODIUM 43mg; CALC 10mg

RECIPE BENEFITS: low-fat; low-sodium

CHOICE INGREDIENT: Oats contain soluble fiber, which can help lower cholesterol and reduce the risk of heart disease. They are low in fat and contain no sodium or preservatives.

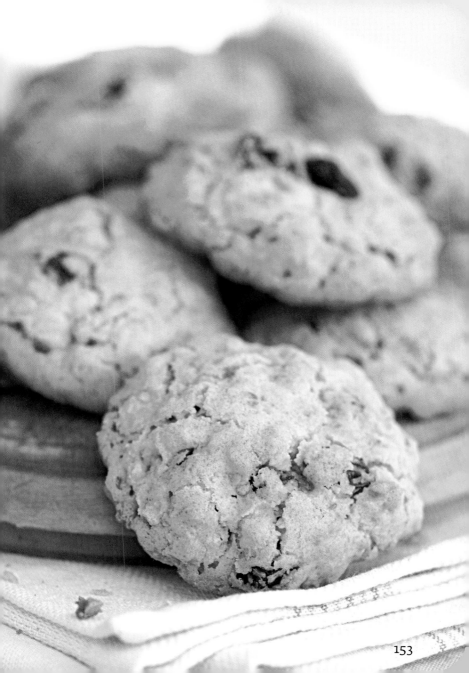

Blueberry Crisp à la Mode

The next time you see a farm stand selling summer-ripe blueberries, make a quick stop. Sample one or two berries to make sure they're juicy and sweet. Then head home to make this comforting dessert. You should have the other ingredients in your pantry. The not-too-sweet flavor comes more from the generous amount of blueberries than from added sugar.

6 **cups blueberries**	$^1/_2$ **cup regular oats**
2 **tablespoons brown sugar**	$^3/_4$ **teaspoon ground cinnamon**
1 **tablespoon all-purpose flour**	$4^1/_2$ **tablespoons chilled butter,**
1 **tablespoon fresh lemon juice**	**cut into small pieces**
3 **ounces all-purpose flour**	2 **cups vanilla low-fat frozen**
(about $^2/_3$ **cup)**	**yogurt**
$^1/_2$ **cup packed brown sugar**	

1. Preheat oven to 375°.

2. Combine first 4 ingredients in a medium bowl; spoon into an 11 x 7–inch baking dish. Weigh or lightly spoon flour into a dry measuring cup; level with a knife. Combine flour, $^1/_2$ cup brown sugar, oats, and cinnamon; cut in butter with a pastry blender or 2 knives until mixture resembles coarse meal. Sprinkle over blueberry mixture. Bake at 375° for 30 minutes or until bubbly. Top each serving with $^1/_4$ cup frozen yogurt. **YIELD:** 8 servings (serving size: $^1/_8$ of crisp).

Note: The topping may also be made in a food processor. Place flour, $^1/_2$ cup brown sugar, oats, and cinnamon in a food processor, and pulse 2 times or until combined. Add butter, and pulse 4 times or until mixture resembles coarse meal.

CALORIES 288; FAT 8.3g (sat 4.8g, mono 2g, poly 0.9g); PROTEIN 4.2g; CARB 52g; FIBER 3.8g; CHOL 22mg; IRON 1.3mg; SODIUM 96mg; CALC 77mg

RECIPE BENEFITS: low-fat; low-sodium

CHOICE INGREDIENT: *Blueberries*

Blueberries are an excellent source of disease-fighting antioxidants that may help prevent cancer and heart disease. Low in calories, high in fiber, and virtually fat-free, blueberries are the perfect sweet and healthy summer treat. Although available year-round, blueberries are best when they're in season and are less expensive then, too. You can freeze them to enjoy months later. Look for firm berries with a silvery frost, and discard any that are shriveled and moldy. Don't wash them until you are ready to use them. Store blueberries in the refrigerator for up to five days.

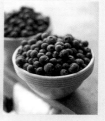

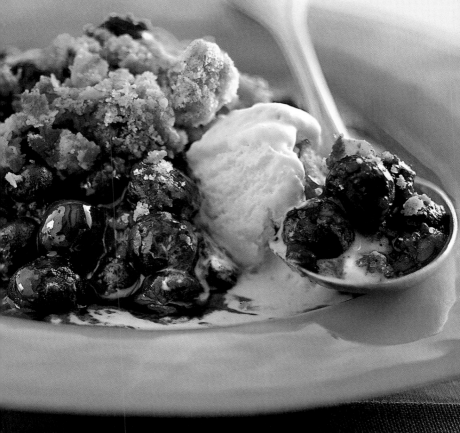

Grilled Nectarines and Plums with Vanilla Bean Syrup

Grilling heightens the fruits' sweetness. Slightly firm fruit will stand up to the heat; if you're using ripe fruit, remove it from the grill a few minutes sooner than directed. Garnish with mint sprigs.

2 cups water
1/3 cup honey
1 (3-inch) vanilla bean, split lengthwise
1/4 cup frozen fat-free whipped topping, thawed
2 tablespoons mascarpone cheese

1 tablespoon honey
4 nectarines, halved and pitted
4 plums, halved and pitted
Cooking spray
2 cups cherries, halved and pitted
2 tablespoons sliced almonds, toasted and chopped

1. Preheat grill.

2. Combine 2 cups water and 1/3 cup honey in a small saucepan over medium-high heat. Scrape seeds from vanilla bean, and add seeds to honey mixture. Discard bean. Bring to a boil. Cook until reduced to 1 1/4 cups (about 15 minutes). Combine whipped topping, cheese, and 1 tablespoon honey, stirring until smooth. Set aside.

3. Lightly coat both sides of nectarines and plums with cooking spray. Place nectarines and plums, cut sides down, on grill rack coated with cooking spray. Grill 2 minutes on each side or until soft. Place 1 nectarine half and 1 plum half in each of 8 shallow bowls. Top each serving with 1/4 cup cherries; drizzle each with 2 tablespoons honey mixture. Spoon 2 teaspoons cheese mixture over each serving; sprinkle each serving with 3/4 teaspoon nuts.

YIELD: 8 servings (serving size: 1 bowl).

CALORIES 173; FAT 4.6g (sat 1.9g, mono 1.6g, poly 0.5g); PROTEIN 2.1g; CARB 33.7g; FIBER 2g; CHOL 9mg; IRON 0.5mg; SODIUM 6mg; CALC 21mg

RECIPE BENEFITS: low-fat; low-sodium

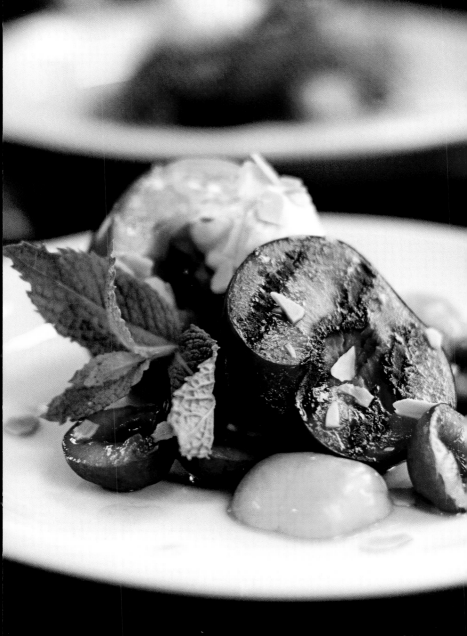

Citrus and Kiwifruit Salad with Pomegranate Seeds and Pistachios

With vibrant orange citrus slices and flecks of jewel-colored pomegranate seeds, this refreshing dish can be served as a dessert or as a side salad.

3 kiwifruit, peeled and sliced (about 1 cup)

4 oranges, peeled and sliced (about 2 cups)

2 red grapefruit, peeled and sectioned (about 2 cups)

1/4 cup pomegranate seeds (about 1 pomegranate)

1 teaspoon orange-flower water (optional)

2 tablespoons coarsely chopped pistachios

1. Divide kiwifruit and oranges evenly among 6 serving bowls; top evenly with grapefruit and pomegranate seeds. Drizzle orange-flower water evenly over fruit, if desired. Sprinkle each serving with 1 teaspoon pistachios. **YIELD:** 6 servings (serving size: about 1 cup).

CALORIES 131; FAT 1.7g (sat 0.2g, mono 0.7g, poly 0.5g); PROTEIN 2.6g; CARB 29.4g; FIBER 4.6g; CHOL 0mg; IRON 0.5mg; SODIUM 3mg; CALC 67mg

RECIPE BENEFITS: low-fat; low-sodium

MAKE-AHEAD TIP: Peel the oranges, kiwifruit, and grapefruit ahead, and refrigerate separately in heavy-duty zip-top plastic bags. Wait until the morning of the day you plan to serve to cut them so they'll retain their sweet juiciness. Seed the pomegranate in advance; refrigerate in a zip-top plastic bag. Spoon the fruit and seeds into individual bowls within an hour of serving; sprinkle with nuts at the last minute.

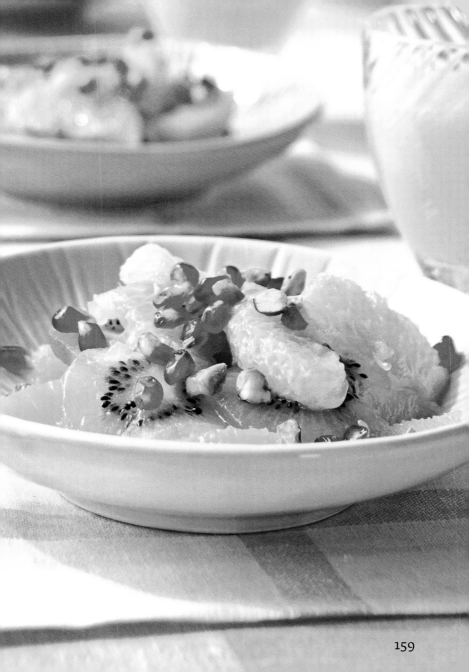

159

Raspberry Frozen Yogurt

This light, refreshing dessert makes an ideal finish for a multicourse meal. Serve with biscotti. Garnish with fresh mint sprigs, if you like.

2 cups vanilla low-fat yogurt
$^1/_2$ cup whole milk
$^1/_4$ cup sugar

1 (10-ounce) package frozen raspberries in light syrup, thawed
Fresh raspberries (optional)

1. Combine first 3 ingredients in a large bowl; stir until sugar dissolves.

2. Place thawed raspberries in a blender; process until smooth. Strain puree through a fine sieve over a bowl. Discard seeds. Add puree to yogurt mixture.

3. Pour raspberry mixture into the freezer can of an ice-cream freezer; freeze according to manufacturer's instructions. Spoon into a freezer-safe container; cover and freeze 1 hour or until firm. Garnish with fresh raspberries, if desired. **YIELD:** 8 servings (serving size: $^1/_2$ cup).

CALORIES 100; FAT 1.3g (sat 0.8g, mono 0.3g, poly 0.1g); PROTEIN 3.8g; CARB 18.6g; FIBER 0.5g; CHOL 5mg; IRON 0.2mg; SODIUM 47mg; CALC 124mg

RECIPE BENEFITS: low-fat; low-sodium

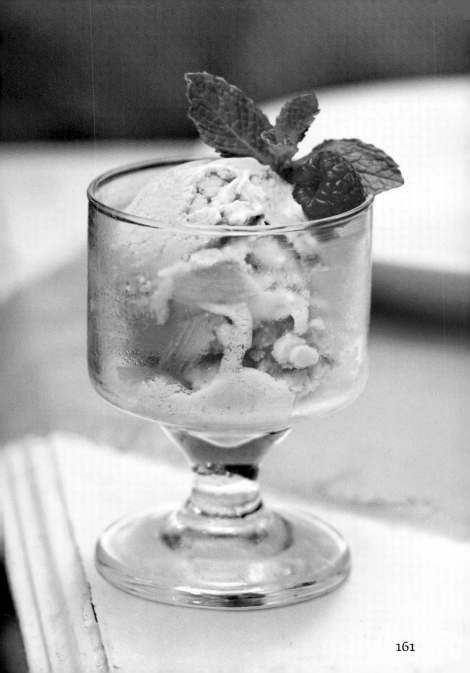

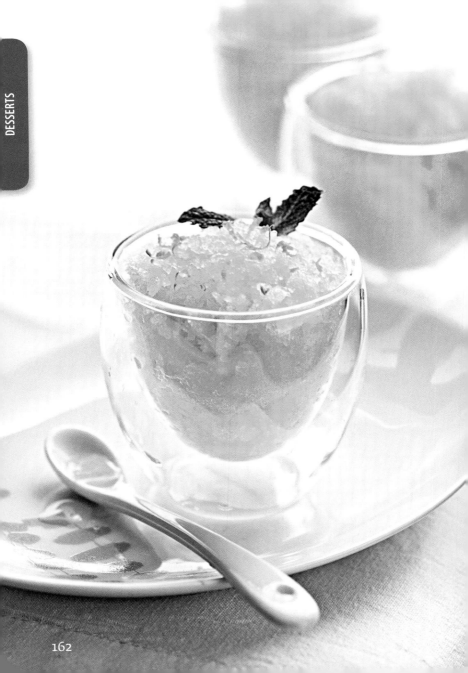

Fresh Orange Sorbet

This sorbet has been a fixture for our Test Kitchens staffers since it was first tested. It is a standby for special occasions.

2½ **cups water**
1 **cup sugar**
Orange rind strips from 2 oranges
2⅔ **cups fresh orange juice**

⅓ **cup fresh lemon juice**
Grated orange rind (optional)
Mint sprigs (optional)

1. Combine 2½ cups water and sugar in a saucepan; bring to a boil. Add rind strips to pan. Reduce heat, and simmer 5 minutes. Strain sugar mixture through a sieve over a bowl, reserving liquid; discard solids. Cool sugar mixture completely.
2. Add orange juice and lemon juice to sugar mixture; stir well. Pour mixture into the freezer can of an ice-cream freezer; freeze according to manufacturer's instructions. Spoon sorbet into a freezer-safe container; cover and freeze 1 hour or until firm. Garnish with grated rind and mint sprigs, if desired. **YIELD:** 12 servings (serving size: ½ cup).

CALORIES 91; FAT 0g; PROTEIN 0.4g; CARB 23.1g; FIBER 0.2g; CHOL 0mg; IRON 0.1mg; SODIUM 1mg; CALC 5mg
RECIPE BENEFITS: fat-free; low-sodium

5 Speedy Fail-Safe Sides

Try these sensational side dishes when time is of the essence.

Parmesan-Chive Mashed Potatoes: Heat 1 (20-ounce) package refrigerated mashed potatoes (such as Simply Potatoes) according to package directions. Stir in $^1/_4$ cup grated fresh Parmesan cheese, 2 tablespoons chopped fresh chives, and $^1/_2$ teaspoon freshly ground black pepper.

Broccoli with Balsamic-Butter Sauce: Place 1 pound trimmed broccoli spears in a microwave-safe dish; add 1 tablespoon water. Cover with plastic wrap; vent. Microwave at HIGH 4 minutes or until crisp-tender; drain. Melt 1 tablespoon butter in a large nonstick skillet over medium-high heat. Add 2 tablespoons finely chopped shallots; sauté 2 minutes. Remove from heat. Stir in 2 tablespoons balsamic vinegar, $^1/_4$ teaspoon salt, and $^1/_4$ teaspoon freshly ground black pepper; drizzle over broccoli.

Oven-Roasted Green Beans: Preheat oven to 475°. Combine 1 pound trimmed green beans, 2 teaspoons olive oil, $^1/_2$ teaspoon salt, and $^1/_8$ teaspoon black pepper. Arrange in a single layer on a baking sheet coated with cooking spray. Bake at 475° for 10 minutes or until tender, turning once. Remove from oven; toss with 2 teaspoons fresh lemon juice.

Sautéed Corn and Tomatoes: Heat a large nonstick skillet over medium-high heat. Coat pan with cooking spray. Add $1^1/_2$ cups frozen whole-kernel corn, thawed; sauté 2 minutes or until tender. Add 1 (1-pound) container grape tomatoes, halved; sauté 1 minute. Add 1 tablespoon sliced fresh basil, $^1/_4$ teaspoon freshly ground black pepper, and $^1/_8$ teaspoon salt; sauté 1 minute or until basil wilts.

Asian Coleslaw: Place 1 cup frozen shelled edamame in a colander, and rinse under cool running water to thaw; drain well. Combine edamame, 4 cups angel hair slaw, $^1/_4$ cup light sesame ginger dressing (such as Newman's Own), and 2 tablespoons chopped fresh cilantro in a large bowl. Toss well.

Nutritional Analysis

How to Use It and Why Glance at the end of any *Cooking Light* recipe, and you'll see how committed we are to helping you make the best of today's light cooking. With chefs, registered dietitians, home economists, and a computer system that analyzes every ingredient, *Cooking Light* gives you authoritative dietary detail like no other magazine. We go to such lengths so you can see how our recipes fit into your healthful eating plan. If you're trying to lose weight, the calorie and fat figures will probably help most. But if you're keeping a close eye on the sodium, cholesterol, and saturated fat in your diet, we provide those numbers, too. And because many women don't get enough iron or calcium, we can help there as well. Finally, there's a fiber analysis for those of us who don't get enough roughage.

Here's a helpful guide to put our nutritional analysis numbers into perspective. Remember, one size doesn't fit all, so take your lifestyle, age, and circumstances into consideration when determining your nutrition needs. For example, pregnant or breast-feeding women need more protein, calories, and calcium. And women older than 50 need 1,200mg of calcium daily—200mg more than the amount recommended for younger women.

In Our Nutritional Analysis, We Use These Abbreviations

sat	saturated fat	**CHOL**	cholesterol
mono	monounsaturated fat	**CALC**	calcium
poly	polyunsaturated fat	**g**	gram
CARB	carbohydrates	**mg**	milligram

Daily Nutrition Guide

	Women Ages 25 to 50	Women over 50	Men over 24
Calories	2,000	2,000 or less	2,700
Protein	50g	50g or less	63g
Fat	65g or less	65g or less	88g or less
Saturated Fat	20g or less	20g or less	27g or less
Carbohydrates	304g	304g	410g
Fiber	25g to 35g	25g to 35g	25g to 35g
Cholesterol	300mg or less	300mg or less	300mg or less
Iron	18mg	8mg	8mg
Sodium	2,300mg or less	1,500mg or less	2,300mg or less
Calcium	1,000mg	1,200mg	1,000mg

Metric Equivalents

The information in the following charts is provided to help cooks outside the United States successfully use the recipes in this book. All equivalents are approximate.

Liquid Ingredients by Volume

¼ tsp	= 1 ml			
½ tsp	= 2 ml			
1 tsp	= 5 ml			
3 tsp	= 1 tbl	= ½ floz	= 15 ml
2 tbls	= ⅛ cup	= 1 floz	= 30 ml
4 tbls	= ¼ cup	= 2 floz	= 60 ml
5⅓ tbls	= ⅓ cup	= 3 floz	= 80 ml
8 tbls	= ½ cup	= 4 floz	= 120 ml
10⅔ tbls	= ⅔ cup	= 5 floz	= 160 ml
12 tbls	= ¾ cup	= 6 floz	= 180 ml
16 tbls	= 1 cup	= 8 floz	= 240 ml
1 pt	= 2 cups	= 16 floz	= 480 ml
1 qt	= 4 cups	= 32 floz	= 960 ml
		33 floz	= 1000 ml	= 1l

Length
(To convert inches to centimeters, multiply the number of inches by 2.5.)

1 in =		2.5 cm
6 in = ½ft	= 15 cm	
12 in = 1ft	= 30 cm	
36 in = 3ft = 1yd	= 90 cm	
40 in =		100 cm = 1m

Dry Ingredients by Weight
(To convert ounces to grams, multiply the number of ounces by 30.)

1 oz	=	¹⁄₁₆ lb	=	30 g
4 oz	=	¼ lb	=	120 g
8 oz	=	½ lb	=	240 g
12 oz	=	¾ lb	=	360 g
16 oz	=	1 lb	=	480 g

Cooking/Oven Temperatures

Fahrenheit	Celsius	Gas Mark
32° F	0° C	
68° F	20° C	
212° F	100° C	
325° F	160° C	3
350° F	180° C	4
375° F	190° C	5
400° F	200° C	6
425° F	220° C	7
450° F	230° C	8

Equivalents for Different Types of Ingredients

Standard Cup	Fine Powder (ex. flour)	Grain (ex. rice)	Granular (ex. sugar)	Liquid Solids (ex. butter)	Liquid (ex. milk)
1	140 g	150 g	190 g	200 g	240 ml
¾	105 g	113 g	143 g	150 g	180 ml
⅔	93 g	100 g	125 g	133 g	160 ml
½	70 g	75 g	95 g	100 g	120 ml
⅓	47 g	50 g	63 g	67 g	80 ml
¼	35 g	38 g	48 g	50 g	60 ml
⅛	18 g	19 g	24 g	25 g	30 ml

Subject Index

Recipe Index

*quick & easy

Fish & Shellfish *(continued)*

*Maple Grilled Salmon, 22
*Pistachio-Crusted Grouper with Lavender Honey
  Sauce, 12
*Sautéed Snapper with Orange-Fennel Salad, 18
*Seared Mahimahi with Edamame Succotash, 15
*Seared Scallops with Warm Fruit Salsa, 41
Sesame Shrimp Salad, 36
Smoky Shrimp and Parmesan-Polenta Cakes, 33
Tuna with Avocado Green Goddess Aïoli, 28

Meatless

Black Bean Soup, 70
*Black Lentil and Couscous Salad, 58
*Bulgur Salad with Edamame and Cherry Tomatoes, 60
*Cavatappi with Arugula Pesto and Grape Tomatoes, 51
Falafel with Avocado Spread, 66
Feta and Green Onion Couscous Cakes over Tomato-Olive
  Salad, 64
Grilled Vegetable Pitas with Goat Cheese and Pesto
  Mayo, 68
Lentil-Edamame Stew, 73
*Pasta with Zucchini and Toasted Almonds, 52
Red Lentil-Rice Cakes with Tomato Salsa, 46
*Sautéed Vegetables and Spicy Tofu, 54
Summer Squash Pizza, 56
White Beans with Roasted Red Pepper and Pesto, 48

Meats

Beef and Beer Chili, 99
*Filet Mignon with Arugula Salad, 83
Grilled Flank Steak Soft Tacos with Avocado-Lime
  Salsa, 77
*Grilled Pork Sliders with Honey BBQ Sauce, 97
*Grilled Pork with Blackberry-Sage Sauce, 91
*Individual Salsa Meat Loaves, 87
*Mongolian Beef, 78
*Pork Chops with Mustard Cream Sauce, 88
*Posole, 100
*Roasted Flank Steak with Olive Oil-Herb Rub, 80
Roasted Pork Tenderloin with Orange and Red Onion
  Salsa, 93
Slow-Cooker Beef Pot Roast, 85
*Warm Spinach Salad with Pork and Pears, 94

Poultry

*Chicken Bulgur Salad, 120
*Chicken Caesar Salad, 123
Chicken, Cashew, and Red Pepper Stir-Fry, 117

Chicken Scaloppine with Sugar Snap Pea, Asparagus,
  and Lemon Salad, 113
*Chicken-Escarole Soup, 132
*Cilantro-Lime Chicken with Avocado Salsa, 109
*Grilled Chicken and Pineapple Sandwiches, 127
Grilled Chicken Thighs with Roasted Grape
  Tomatoes, 119
*Mediterranean Turkey Burgers, 128
Peanut-Crusted Chicken with Pineapple Salsa, 114
*Sesame Brown Rice Salad with Shredded Chicken
  and Peanuts, 107
White Bean and Turkey Chili, 135

Salads

*Black Lentil and Couscous Salad, 58
*Bulgur Salad with Edamame and Cherry Tomatoes, 60
*Chicken Bulgur Salad, 120
*Chicken Caesar Salad, 123
*Sesame Brown Rice Salad with Shredded Chicken
  and Peanuts, 107
Sesame Shrimp Salad, 36
*Warm Spinach Salad with Pork and Pears, 94

Sandwiches

Falafel with Avocado Spread, 66
*Grilled Chicken and Pineapple Sandwiches, 127
*Grilled Pork Sliders with Honey BBQ Sauce, 97
Grilled Vegetable Pitas with Goat Cheese and Pesto
  Mayo, 68
*Mediterranean Turkey Burgers, 128

Soups & Stews

Beef and Beer Chili, 99
Black Bean Soup, 70
*Chicken-Escarole Soup, 132
Lentil-Edamame Stew, 73
*Posole, 100
White Bean and Turkey Chili, 135

Sides

*Asian Coleslaw, 164
*Broccoli with Balsamic-Butter Sauce, 164
Herbed Sweet Potato Fries, 96
Jack and Red Pepper Quesadillas, 98
*Oven-Roasted Green Beans, 164
*Parmesan-Chive Mashed Potatoes, 164
*Sautéed Corn and Tomatoes, 164

quick & easy